Get Through

MRCOphth Part 3: EMQs

Sharmina R A Khan BSc MBBS MRCOphth
Specialist Registrar South Thames

Ourania Frangouli MD MRCOphth
Specialist Registrar North Thames

The ROYAL
SOCIETY *of*
MEDICINE

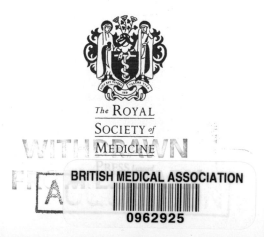

Published by the Royal Society of Medicine Press Ltd
1 Wimpole Street, London W1G 0AE, UK
Tel: +44 (0)20 7290 2921
Fax: +44 (0)20 7290 2929
Email: publishing@rsm.ac.uk
Website: www.rsmpress.co.uk

British Library Cataloguing in Publication Data
A catalogue record for this book is available from the British Library

ISBN 1-85315-609-4

Distribution in Europe and Rest of World:

Marston Book Services Ltd
PO Box 269
Abingdon
Oxon OX14 4YN, UK
Tel: +44 (0)1235 465500
Fax: +44 (0)1235 465555
Email: direct.order@marston.co.uk

Distribution in the USA and Canada:

Royal Society of Medicine Press Ltd
c/o BookMasters Inc
30 Amberwood Parkway
Ashland, OH 44805, USA
Tel: +1 800 247 6553/+1 800 266 5564
Fax: +1 419 281 6883
Email: order@bookmasters.com

Distribution in Australia and New Zealand:

Elsevier Australia
30–52 Smidmore Street
Marrikville NSW 2204, Australia
Tel: +61 2 9349 5811
Fax: +61 2 9349 5911
Email: service@elsevier.com.au

Designed and typeset by SR Nova, India
Printed and bound by Bell & Bain, Glasgow

Contents

Preface

This book is designed to aid trainee Ophthalmologists in their preparation for the Part 3 Membership examination of the Royal College of Ophthalmologists' Extended Matching Questions (EMQs) paper.

The questions in this book do not comprehensively cover the entire syllabus and you should refer to the college curriculum. The questions will go through differential diagnosis, investigations and the management of both common and uncommon clinical scenarios.

The clinical scenarios are based on our reading, teaching sessions and clinical experience as Senior House Officers at Moorfields Eye Hospital, and as Specialist Registrars in North and South Thames Deaneries. We would like to thank our colleagues for their kindness and helpful suggestions during the preparation of the manuscript, in particular: Adam Bates, John Brookes and Niaz Islam.

Sharmina Khan and Ourania Frangouli

Chapter 1

Adnexal and Orbit – EMQs

- This chapter consists of 114 extended matching questions.
- Questions consist of a theme, a list of options, an instruction and a variable number of clinical situations.
- For each of the clinical situations, you should choose the **single most likely option** according to the instruction.
- It is possible for one option to be the answer to more than one of the clinical situations.

Theme: Lid lesions I

Options
A   Papilloma
B   Pedunculated seborrhoeic keratosis
C   Molluscum contagiosum
D   Cutaneous horn
E   Syringoma
F   Keratoacanthoma

For each of the clinical scenarios below, select the single most likely diagnosis from the list above. Each option may be used once, more than once or not at all.

1.   A 10-year-old boy presents in the eye casualty with a pearly white lesion on his lower eyelid. His mother noticed it only in the past 3 weeks. It has started to enlarge slightly. The eye is red and inflamed on this side. On slit-lamp examination there appears to be a central keratin plug that gives the lesion an umbilicated appearance.

2.   A 40-year-old gentleman attends the eye clinic. He has been referred urgently by his GP for a lesion on his left upper lid that has rapidly grown over the past month. He is asymptomatic and the lesion has spontaneously almost completely resolved but he is currently bothered by the cosmetic appearance. Biomicroscopy shows an isolated dome-shaped nodule with a keratotic plug in the centre, of red to light brown in colour.

3.   You are examining a 39-year-old man. He has multiple lesions in the lower lids bilaterally. He explains that they were flat initially but gradually with time they became more pigmented and slightly 'warty' in appearance. He also mentions that he has similar lesions in his upper arms.

Theme: Lids

Options
A Chalazion
B Hordeolum
C Floppy eyelid syndrome
D Chronic papillary conjunctivitis
E Sebaceous adenocarcinoma
F Apocrine hydrocystoma

For each of the clinical scenarios below, select the single most likely diagnosis from the list above. Each option may be used once, more than once or not at all.

4. A 34-year-old man with sleep apnoea is examined in a general clinic. He complains of a longstanding non-specific irritation of both eyes. This becomes worse at night time. The palpebral conjunctiva has a velvety appearance and there is tarsal papillary conjunctivitis. He is also obese. He is listed for a horizontal lid tightening procedure.

5. A 65-year-old gentleman attends the eye casualty. You note that he has multiple attendances in the past few months with unilateral blepharitis. He has a record of a minor operation in his left lower lid. He complains that the cyst in his lower lid keeps recurring despite adequate treatment. On examination he has a small nodular lesion that is slightly inflamed. The lid margin is also erythematous on this side.

6. In the minor operations clinic you examine a 24-year-old female patient. She complains of a cyst in her upper eyelid that has been intermittently inflamed for the past few months. She explains that initially it was so inflamed that the whole eyelid was oedematous and she had a course of oral antibiotics by her GP.

Theme: Lid lesions II

Options
A   Haemangioma of the eyelid
B   Port-wine stain
C   Keratoacanthoma
D   Strawberry naevus
E   Plexiform neurofibroma
F   Pyogenic granuloma

For each of the clinical scenarios below, select the single most likely diagnosis from the list above. Each option may be used once, more than once or not at all.

7.   You are called to examine a newborn baby because the paediatricians have noticed a well-demarcated, subcutaneous pink patch involving the left side of face over the baby's forehead and cheek. The overlying skin is slightly swollen. The baby has also had a few fits.

8.   A 10-year-old girl has been referred by her GP to the paediatric ophthalmology clinic. The GP is concerned about unilateral ptosis. There is a lesion on the left upper lid giving the lid an S-shaped pattern. Your consultant asks you to examine her iris and optic nerve and skin. You note that she has been under the paediatricians for a long time.

9.   You are in the clinic. The paediatricians have referred a 12-month-old girl because of a red-purple lesion under the right eyebrow. The father has noticed it for sometime but it has increased in size over the past 4 months. The mother says she is not too bothered by its appearance at the moment but relatives and friends comment on it especially when the baby is crying. She shows you the child's right arm, which has a similar small red spot.

Theme: Neoplasms of the lid I

Options
A   Actinic keratosis
B   Keratoacanthoma
C   Lentigo maligna
D   Basal cell carcinoma
E   Squamous cell carcinoma
F   Sebaceous gland carcinoma

For each of the clinical scenarios below, select the single most likely diagnosis from the list above. Each option may be used once, more than once or not at all.

10.   You have excised a lesion from the right upper lid of a 65-year-old gentleman. He has spent most of his life in Mediterranean countries. The lesion has irregular borders and is darkly pigmented. The histopathologist contacts you and informs you that it is a malignant melanoma deeply invading the surrounding ocular tissues. The patient says he had noticed many years prior to that a dark 'stain' on the skin of that area. Which one of the above is it?

11.   A 40-year-old Australian gentleman has attended the clinic. On examination he appears to have multiple light brown lesions on the left cheek and brow. They are slightly elevated, hyperkeratotic and scaling. He has noticed them in the past couple of years. You explain the nature of the lesions but warn him that they may develop into which of the above?

12.   An 85-year-old man presents in the eye casualty. He complains of mild binocular horizontal diplopia at dextroversion. He also mentions a small ulcerated nodular lump on the medial canthus and caruncle of the left eye. He can't remember exactly for how long this has been there. On questioning he mentions that he had a similar lesion removed from his nose by the dermatologists a few years ago. There is no lymphadenopathy on palpation of the submandibular and pre-auricular nodes. What is the most likely clinical diagnosis?

Theme: Neoplasms of the lid II

Options
A   Malignant melanoma
B   Kaposi sarcoma
C   Pigmented BCC
D   Merkel cell tumour
E   Sebaceous adenocarcinoma
F   Squamous cell carcinoma

For each of the clinical scenarios below, select the single most likely diagnosis from the list above. Each option may be used once, more than once or not at all.

13. You are examining a 74-year-old woman in the clinic. She has a history of a crusty lesion on her left upper eyelid. She has been already referred twice in the minor ops clinic directly by the GP and had shave biopsies. The pathology reports have shown only mild inflammatory changes. You book her for another biopsy and you discuss with the pathologist and ask for lipid (oil red O) stains this time. What is it that you are suspecting?

14. You are contacting the pathologist after excision of a lid lesion prior to consulting a patient. You particularly want to find out about the tumour thickness. What neoplasm are you talking about?

15. An elderly lady had an excisional biopsy of a non-pigmented fleshy tumour causing distortion of her right upper eyelid. The pathology report has ruled out a SCC but it confirms a very rare, highly malignant neoplasm. This is most likely a ... ?

Theme: Treating lid lesions

Options

A   Radiation
B   Cryotherapy
C   Excision and lateral cantholysis
D   Refer to tertiary centre for excision guided by Moh's technique
E   Excision and direct closure
F   Enucleation

For each of the clinical scenarios below, select the single most likely treatment from the list above. Each option may be used once, more than once or not at all.

16.   A 91-year-old lady has been diagnosed with a left medial canthus BCC that is also in close proximity to the lower punctum. Despite having been counselled about the nature of the lesion and the risks, she refuses to have surgery as she feels she is too old to go through another operation. Which alternative treatment modality would you offer this elderly lady?

17.   A 70-year-old gentleman attends his follow-up in the eye clinic. He has a history of a BCC excised from his left lower lid 3 years ago. It was a very small lesion occupying less than 25% of the lid margin. For the past year he has noticed a diffuse lesion over the caruncle of the same eye. This has been growing gradually. You look back at the notes and find the initial histopathology report that mentions that the original lesion was excised with 'narrowly clear' margins. How would you manage this patient?

18.   You are in the operating theatre. A 55-year-old lady has a small BCC in the lateral third of her lower eyelid. After excising it with clear margins you are left with a defect which is around 25% of the lid margin. There is no lid laxity and the skin is quite tight and under tension. How do you decide to repair this defect?

Theme: Surgical procedures

Options
A   Tenzel flap
B   Excision and direct closure
C   Hughes flap and skin graft
D   Excision and canthotomy
E   Burrow's triangles
F   Glabellar flap

For each of the clinical scenarios below, select the single most likely procedure from the list above. Each option may be used once, more than once or not at all.

19. You are operating on a 72-year-old man. He has had a two-stage procedure for a large lower lid SCC. The defect you have to repair in the left lower lid is about 75%. The right eye is amblyopic with VA of counting fingers. Which of the above techniques would you decide to use?

20. The oculoplastic surgeon is repairing the skin after removal of a right medial canthal BCC in an 80-year-old lady. The defect is extending above the nose. Which of the above techniques would be indicated?

21. After a two-stage excision of BCC involving the lower lid of a 70-year-old man, the anterior and posterior lamella of about 85% of the lower eyelid had to be sacrificed. The patient is pseudophakic in the other eye with visual acuity of 6/9. Which of the above techniques would give the best cosmetic and functional result for this patient?

Theme: Surgical interventions

Options
A   Cutler–Beard reconstruction
B   Glabellar flap
C   Semicircular flap
D   'Laissez-faire'
E   Direct closure
F   O-Z flap

For each of the clinical scenarios below, select the single most likely procedure from the list above. Each option may be used once, more than once or not at all.

22.   At the reconstruction stage of a two-stage procedure for an extensive upper lid SCC of a 74-year-old lady, you are left with a defect involving almost 100% of the upper eyelid margin. You would have to take a conjunctival flap from the lower lid. What is the name of this procedure?

23.   The remaining defect is circular and there is significant skin laxity around it. Which technique would give best results functionally and cosmetically?

24.   You are left with a medial upper lid defect that is very small (<25%) and involving the lid margin. There is enough lid laxity. What would you choose to do?

Theme: Eyelid and canalicular trauma

Options
A Primary repair of lid laceration as soon as possible and ptosis surgery as secondary procedure
B Immediate repair of any lid lacerations and brow suspension at one stage
C Clean, check tetanus status, oral metronidazole, repair anterior and posterior limb
D Primary repair in a list the next day
E Anterior and posterior lamellar grafts
F Subcuticular technique for repair

For each of the clinical scenarios below, select the single most likely treatment from the list above. Each option may be used once, more than once or not at all.

25. A young patient presents in the eye casualty out of hours with a dog bite involving the upper and lower lid at the area of the medial canthus. What is the management plan?

26. You are in the eye casualty. A 21-year-old man has been brought in after being assaulted with a broken bottle. You examine the globe carefully. He has a large full thickness laceration in the upper lid and the whole lid is chemotic with signs of a possible traumatic ptosis. How do you plan surgery for this young man?

27. You are on-call and asked by the paediatric registrar to examine a 3-year-old child who has been involved in an RTA. The child is otherwise stable but has significant bruising in her left upper lid and severe traumatic ptosis. The child has already been in hospital for 4 days. You discuss the management with your consultant. What is the most likely decision?

Theme: Canalicular procedures

Options
A   Canalicular intubation technique
B   Repair and marsupialization
C   Primary canalicular DCR with intubation
D   DCR with intubation
E   DCR only
F   Lid margin apposition

For each of the clinical scenarios below, select the single most likely treatment from the list above. Each option may be used once, more than once or not at all.

28.   A 10-year-old boy presents with trauma to his left medial canthus. On slit-lamp examination it is obvious that the lower and upper canaliculi are lacerated. What type of surgical repair would be indicated in this case?

29.   A 25-year-old man has an extensive laceration in the medial canthus and the side of his nose. There is a large deep wound. After cleaning the wound and careful observation you feel that the injury has involved the lacrimal sac and possibly the canaliculi and common canaliculus. As this is a young patient what would you suggest to ensure the best functional outcome?

30.   A 58-year-old gentleman has a laceration in the right medial lower lid margin. There is a laceration of the canaliculus. The upper canaliculus is intact. He cares for his disabled wife and is unable to spend a lot of time in hospital appointments or travel to tertiary centres. What surgical solution would you choose in his case?

Theme: Cicatricial lid malpositions

Options
A   Z-plasty
B   Skin grafting
C   Dermis–fat graft
D   Lateral canthal sling
E   Lazy-T procedure
F   Khunt–Symanovsky

For each of the clinical scenarios below, select the single most likely procedure from the list above. Each option may be used once, more than once or not at all.

31.   A 48-year-old patient attends the outpatients department. He has been referred by his GP for constant epiphora and irritation from his right eye. Five years prior to that he had an injury to his right lower lid which was repaired at a general A&E department by the casualty officer. On examination the lid is slightly turning outwards and there is an obvious vertical scar on the lower lid. You advise him regarding surgery for correction. What procedure would you decide to use?

32.   You are assessing the patients for the afternoon theatre list. You are examining a 50-year-old lady with a history of previous burn in her left lower lid. You notice there is significant shortening of the anterior lamella. What procedure do you have to advise this patient of?

33.   A 50-year-old female patient with OCP has been referred. Her systemic condition is stable on immunosuppressant drugs. She has significant cicatricial changes especially in the upper lid sulcus despite the systemic and topical medication. As she is stable she would like to consider surgery to improve her ocular condition. Which of the above solutions is suitable in her case?

Theme: Eyelid malpositions

Options
A   Acute spastic entropion
B   Congenital entropion
C   Congenital epiblepharon
D   Epiblepharon
E   Blepharophimosis
F   Congenital distichiasis

For each of the clinical scenarios below, select the single most likely diagnosis from the list above. Each option may be used once, more than once or not at all.

34.   You are asked by the SCBU paediatric registrar to examine a premature baby. His left eye appears to have been irritated since birth and he does not want to open it. The SPR feels there might be a corneal opacity in the affected eye. There are no other corneal or anterior segment abnormalities on examination. What is the most likely diagnosis?

35.   The paediatric consultant refers a 4-week-old child. The reason for referral is that the baby's father has been under the ophthalmic department in the past as he suffers with bilateral ptosis, telecanthus and epicanthus inversus. On examination the baby also has a poorly developed nasal bridge and hypertelorism. What is the most likely diagnosis?

36.   A 4-year-old boy attends the outpatients department. You note from his history that he had multiple sessions of electrolysis in the past. What was the reason for that?

Theme: Entropion I

Options
A   Anterior lamellar repositioning
B   Tarsal wedge resection
C   Everting sutures
D   Quickert's procedure
E   Jones' procedure
F   Tarsal dissection +/– mucous membrane graft (MMG)

For each of the clinical scenarios below, select the single most likely treatment from the list above. Each option may be used once, more than once or not at all.

37. A 34-year-old man with a history of Stevens–Johnson syndrome comes to see you. He is systemically stable at the moment but suffers with constant epiphora and redness of his left lower lid. He would like to discuss surgery for correcting his lower lid position. What is the appropriate surgical method?

38. An elderly lady attends her clinic follow-up. She complains that despite previous multiple electrolysis treatments her upper eyelid lashes still rub on her cornea causing her constant discomfort. On close inspection you realize that it is the lid position causing the problem. You list her for surgical repair. Which of the above is the indicated procedure in her case?

39. A 68-year-old man has a longstanding right lower lid entropion. On examination there is significant horizontal laxity and looking back through his notes you can see that he has already had everting sutures and a Wies procedure for correction in the past. He would like another operation. What is the preferable surgical method to follow?

Theme: Entropion II

Options
A   Full thickness pentagon excision and direct closure
B   Khunt–Symanovsky
C   Lateral canthal sling
D   Tarsoconjunctival diamond excision
E   Gold weight implantation
F   Plication of medial canthal tendon

For each of the clinical scenarios below, select the single most likely treatment from the list above. Each option may be used once, more than once or not at all.

40.   A 76-year-old lady is assessed before an operating session. She has an involutional right lower lid ectropion. On examination there is downward sag of the lower lid margin centrally. When the lid is pulled away from the eye it does not resume its normal position spontaneously. There is no canthal laxity. However there is a significant amount of excess skin. What is the surgical procedure you decide to perform?

41.   Again you are assessing a patient for theatre. He has an involutional ectropion. This time there is horizontal lid laxity and significant lateral laxity. What would be the procedure of choice?

42.   A 50-year-old patient has a moderate right lower lid ectropion. On careful examination, the ectropion is mainly medially. There is no horizontal laxity and the medial canthus is intact. What is the quickest and simplest procedure you can carry out for this patient?

Theme: Adnexal clinic I

Options
A   Cicatricial ectropion
B   Paralytic ectropion
C   Symblepharon with superior fornix shortening
D   Involutional ectropion
E   Mechanical ectropion
F   Blepharochalasis

For each of the clinical scenarios below, select the single most likely diagnosis from the list above. Each option may be used once, more than once or not at all.

43.   A patient attends her clinic follow-up. She is stable at the moment and comments that her left eye is much more comfortable. Her notes are missing. On examination you notice a scar on the skin on the lateral aspect of her eyelid and around the lateral canthus. There is also a firm, palpable mass on her upper eyelid. It is obvious that she has had procedures for correction of which type of ectropion?

44.   A 58-year-old man attends his postoperative follow-up 1 week after his operation. He has had a surgical procedure on his left lower lid. There is also a pressure pad in front of his left ear. What type of ectropion did he have?

45.   A young man attends the eye casualty. He complains that his lower lid is very floppy and lax and has been turning out for the past 2 weeks. On examination he has a few large cysts involving the lid margin. There is also some conjunctival chemosis. This is a case of . . . ?

Theme: Ptosis I

Options
A   Congenital myogenic ptosis
B   Muscular dystrophy
C   Blepharophimosis
D   Marcus Gunn jaw winking
E   Congenital Horner's syndrome
F   Neurogenic ptosis

For each of the clinical scenarios below, select the single most likely diagnosis from the list above. Each option may be used once, more than once or not at all.

46.   You are examining a 3-week-old baby. He has a slightly ptotic eyelid on the left side. The left palpebral aperture is much lower than the right. Levator function is about 5 mm. The mother mentions that the ptosis improves slightly when the baby is lying flat and breastfeeding. What is the most likely diagnosis?

47.   A 2-year-old child attends the clinic. He has moderate bilateral ptosis. Levator function is 7 mm on the right and 6 mm on the left side. You note he has a larger fold on the lower lid compared to the upper lid. There is a mild ectropion on the lower lid of the left eye. There is definitely an abnormal nasal bridge and the medial canthi look slightly displaced. What is the diagnosis?

48.   A 3-year-old child has been referred by his doctor for a second opinion. He has a droopy eyelid on the right side and a small convergent squint that he controls by wearing his hypermetropic prescription. Visual acuities are 6/6 in the right eye and 6/5 in the left eye. Parents say they had no major concerns up to this date as the ptosis is not affecting his vision. On slit-lamp examination you notice the iris is of slightly lighter colour on the right side. What is the most likely diagnosis?

Theme: Ptosis II

Options
A   Myasthenia gravis
B   Third nerve palsy
C   Horner's syndrome
D   Myotonic dystrophy
E   Acquired myogenic ptosis
F   Pseudoptosis

For each of the clinical scenarios below, select the single most likely diagnosis from the list above. Each option may be used once, more than once or not at all.

49.   A 70-year-old gentleman is examined in the clinic. He complains of intermittent double vision for the past few months. He also says that his eyes feel heavier towards the end of the day and his wife has noticed his left lid becomes slightly droopy. Orthoptic examination on the day showed only mild exophoria. His orbicularis on the left side is weak. What is the diagnosis you have to exclude?

50.   The physicians have asked you for a second opinion on a 55-year-old gentleman who has been seen in the eye clinic before with bilateral ptosis and at the time he refused surgical repair. His has moderate bilateral ptosis and keeps his chin raised in order to compensate for it. His speech appears to be a bit slurred. He tells you he has been bald since the age of 30. When asking his family history he tells you that he has two daughters aged 20 and 25. His 25-year-old daughter has had bilateral cataract extractions. What is the diagnosis you suspect?

51.   A patient has been referred for cataract extraction. You note that he has a droopy eyelid on the left side. Eyelid position is normal on examination. Orbicularis power is normal. Levator function is 13 mm on the left and 14 mm on the right side. He tells you this does not bother him. His left eye has been like that since he had an eye injury 20 years ago and a fracture in the bones surrounding the eye, which at the time was not repaired. This is a case of ...?

Theme: Ptosis III

Options

A   Simple congenital myogenic ptosis
B   Blepharophimosis
C   Oculopharyngeal dystrophy
D   Congenital ocular fibrosis syndrome
E   Kearns–Sayre syndrome
F   Aberrant regeneration

For each of the clinical scenarios below, select the single most likely diagnosis from the list above. Each option may be used once, more than once or not at all.

52.   You are examining a 2-year-old child in the clinic. He has bilateral ptosis more on the left side. He keeps his chin up. His levator function is 4 mm in the left eye and 9 mm on the right side. On the left side the skin crease is absent and there is lid lag on downgaze. There is mild lagophthalmos on the left. His left eye is amblyopic. This is a case of . . . ?

53.   The neurologists ask you to examine a 17-year-old inpatient. He presented with cerebellar ataxia and muscle weakness. His ECG shows heat block and he has mild ptosis. They want you to check his fundi as well. What is the possible diagnosis?

54.   You are examining a 30-year-old woman. She has severe ptosis. Levator function is 4 mm in the right eye and 3 mm in the left eye. She has external ophthalmoplegia which has not changed in the past 4 years. The eyes are deviated downwards and she has a chin-up head posture to help her. When she tries to look up the eyes converge. Her father had a similar condition. What is the diagnosis?

Theme: Adnexal clinic II

Options
A   Brow ptosis
B   Dermatochalasis
C   Blepharochalasis
D   Blepharospasm
E   Pseudoptosis
F   Brow spasm

For each of the clinical scenarios below, select the single most likely option from the list above. Each option may be used once, more than once or not at all.

55. A 20-year-old woman has come to see you in the clinic. She complains of intermittent swelling of her right eyelid. She is also bothered by the cosmetic appearance of her eyelid as there is a lot of lax and redundant skin both on the upper and lower lids giving her right eye an 'aged' appearance. The skin is very thin and sensitive. What is the most likely diagnosis?

56. Endoscopic, coronal, direct, midforehead and internal approach refer to surgical procedures carried out for ...?

57. An elderly female patient is referred to you for ptosis surgery. She complains her lids feel tired all the time and that she has a defect in her upper visual field bilaterally. On examination her palpebral apertures are almost equal: 11 mm. Her levator function is 14 mm on the right and 13 mm on the left. There is some prolapse of orbital fat bilaterally and there is a lot of loose skin on the temporal aspect of both eyelids. She complains of constant brow ache. You explain to her she does not need ptosis surgery. Her problem is ...?

Theme: Ptosis surgery

Options

A   Levator resection
B   Aponeurosis advancement
C   Brow suspension with autologous fascia lata
D   Brow suspension with Mersilene mesh
E   Aponeurosis tuck
F   Fasanella–Servat procedure

For each of the clinical scenarios below, select the single most likely procedure from the list above. Each option may be used once, more than once or not at all.

58. A patient with Horner's syndrome wishes to have surgical repair of his ptosis. What is the procedure indicated?

59. A 3-year-old child with blepharophimosis syndrome and severe ptosis is at risk of amblyopia especially in the right eye. You refer him to the paediatric oculoplastic surgeon. You explain to the parents the procedure required and the risks involved. What surgical procedure do you counsel them about?

60. A 70-year-old gentleman had a third nerve palsy associated with a posterior communicating artery aneurysm. 18 months later he is stable and he has had squint surgery. He wishes to have surgery to correct his ptosis now. His levator function is 2 mm. What procedure is appropriate in this case of neurogenic ptosis?

Theme: Postoperative management of ptosis surgery

Options

A   Immediate surgical lowering
B   Massage lid and put in traction for 3 months, then redo surgery after
    6 months if no improvement
C   Bilateral redo surgery preferably with autogenous material
D   Tighten bands immediately
E   Release bands as soon as possible
F   Skin crease reformation

For each of the clinical scenarios below, select the single most likely treatment from the list above. Each option may be used once, more than once or not at all.

61.   A child comes for his follow-up visit a week after bilateral brow suspension with Mersilene mesh for congenital ptosis. His right upper lid is significantly overcorrected. His mother says it is very difficult to use his postoperative drops. The right eye looks red and irritated. What is the appropriate course of action?

62.   A 74-year-old gentleman attends his clinic follow-up 1 month after aponeurosis repair. He is happy with the height of his upper eyelid, but he feels that the lid is turning in and the lashes are at a lower position and rub on the cornea causing foreign body sensation. You examine the lid carefully; this problem was not there before the operation. You decide to take him back to theatre. What surgical solution do you offer him?

63.   A 5-year-old child attends her follow-up 1 year after brow suspension. She has a late droop especially in the right eye. What is the option?

Theme: Congenital eyelid anomalies

Options
A   Blepharophimosis
B   Epiblepharon
C   Congenital entropion
D   Congenital coloboma
E   Congenital distichiasis
F   Ankyloblepharon

For each of the clinical scenarios below, select the single most likely diagnosis from the list above. Each option may be used once, more than once or not at all.

64.   A young man has Stevens–Johnson syndrome. His eyelids have significant scarring and they have fused together laterally in the right eye. This is a condition called ...?

65.   A 2-month-old baby is brought in to the clinic. His eyelids are turning inwards to the point that the skin is in contact with the eye. When you examine him you pull the skin back and the lid margin appears to be in good position. The baby has ...?

66.   The neonatal SPR asks you to examine a premature baby. The baby has a facial cleft syndrome. What do you expect you may find?

Theme: Lacrimal apparatus

Options
A Nasolacrimal duct obstruction
B Dacryocystocele
C Lacrimal fistula
D Encephalocele
E Lacrimal sac tumour
F Dacryocystitis

For each of the clinical scenarios below, select the single most likely diagnosis from the list above. Each option may be used once, more than once or not at all.

67. A 68-year-old gentleman complains of multiple episodes of swelling over his right lacrimal sac. He has recently noticed a bloody discharge as well. On examination there is a firm palpable mass. Your consultant decides to order a CT scan. What is he thinking of?

68. You are examining a newborn baby. She has a prominent cystic mass above the medial canthal tendon since birth. You tell the parents you would like to arrange more investigations with the help of the paediatricians before intervening surgically. What are you thinking about?

69. A 1-year-old is referred by her GP. The mother has noticed a small hole on the medial part of her lid. She sometimes notices discharge and tears coming out. On examination she has a small opening inferonasal to the lower punctum. The most likely diagnosis is ...?

Theme: Lacrimal system surgery

Options
A   DCR
B   cDCR with intubation
C   Intubation of canalicular system
D   Lester Jones tube
E   Massage of nasolacrimal duct
F   Syringing and probing

For each of the clinical scenarios below, select the single most likely treatment from the list above. Each option may be used once, more than once or not at all.

70.   A 69-year-old lady with OCP is planned to have surgery for punctual and canalicular stenosis. Which of the above should be avoided?

71.   You are syringing the lacrimal system of a patient in the clinic. After entering the lower canaliculus, the cannula reaches a hard stop. On injecting saline, there is failure of the saline to reach the patient's nasopharynx. There is some regurgitation of purulent saline from the upper punctum. What is the procedure you will offer this patient?

72.   Again on syringing a patient's lacrimal apparatus, the cannula initially reaches a soft stop. There is reflux through the upper canaliculus. You decide to order a DCG. What is the procedure that will be most likely needed?

Theme: Orbit

Options
A   Orbital cellulitis
B   Phycomycosis
C   Orbital pseudotumour
D   Cavernous sinus thrombosis
E   Sarcoidosis
F   Wegener's granulomatosis

For each of the clinical scenarios below, select the single most likely diagnosis from the list above. Each option may be used once, more than once or not at all.

73. You are asked to see an inpatient who is systemically unwell. The patient has a frozen globe, proptosis and fundoscopy shows a central retinal artery occlusion. The patient is a poorly controlled diabetic and has a 2-week history of sinusitis. What is the most likely diagnosis?

74. You are examining a 40-year-old female patient in eye casualty. She has presented with sudden onset of bilateral proptosis. Her lacrimal gland on the right side appears to be enlarged and inflamed. On questioning she tells you that she has always been quite short of breath. You are ordering a CT scan and a chest X-ray. What diagnosis do you suspect?

75. A 67-year-old gentleman presents with sudden onset of proptosis and loss of vision. He is feeling unwell and had renal problems recently. He has external ophthalmoplegia. He has severe intraocular inflammation and the fundus is not visible. B-scan ultrasonography shows a characteristic 'T-sign'. His CT scan is normal. He is admitted under the medics. What is a possible diagnosis?

Theme: Lid lesions I

Options
A   Dermoid cyst
B   Ruptured dermoid cyst
C   Dermolipoma
D   Mucocele
E   Encephalocele
F   Capillary haemangioma

For each of the clinical scenarios below, select the single most likely diagnosis from the list above. Each option may be used once, more than once or not at all.

76.   A 15-year-old girl attends the clinic. She has noticed a yellowish pink lesion at the superotemporal globe. On examination there is a soft mass deep to the conjunctiva. In CT scan the lacrimal gland is intact and in place. There is a mass with fat density. You decide to do nothing about this lesion. What is it?

77.   A 2-year-old child presents with sudden onset of proptosis. There is a lesion in the medial aspect of the orbit which has gradually increased in size and is causing amblyopia of about five dioptres of astigmatism. There is a bluish discoloration of the skin. The child has a CT scan which shows a well-defined mass which enhances with contrast. The orbital surgeons perform a biopsy and rhabdomyosarcoma is ruled out. What is the most likely diagnosis then?

78.   A mother with her 1-year-old child attends the paediatric ophthalmology clinic. The child has a soft mobile mass along the superior temporal rim of his left orbit. The mother insists it has been present since birth. There are no other concerns regarding the systemic health of this child and no other ocular abnormalities are detected during examination. You decide to follow this up at present. This is a case of ...?

Theme: Orbital lesions I

Options
A   Cavernous haemangioma
B   Capillary haemangioma
C   Lymphangioma
D   Schwannoma
E   Lymphoma
F   Haemangiopericytoma

For each of the clinical scenarios below, select the single most likely diagnosis from the list above. Each option may be used once, more than once or not at all.

79.   A 12-year-old girl presents with proptosis and recurrent orbital pain. On examination there is an area of superior subconjunctival haemorrhage. CT scan shows a mass which is rather diffuse and heterogenous. A subsequent MRI of the orbits shows that the mass is hyperintense on T1 and strongly hyperintense on T2. There is a possible area of blood and fluid. As the proptosis is compromising the girl's visual acuity you refer her for drainage. The diagnosis is ... ?

80.   A 52-year-old woman has been referred by her doctor. She has a slowly developing axial proptosis in the right eye. Apart from that she has no visual symptoms. Fundal examination shows choroidal folds. She has had a CT scan which reveals a well-defined encapsulated intraconal mass that is displacing the optic nerve medially. On MRI the lesion is isointense on T1 and hyperintense on T2. It is markedly enhanced with gadolinium. You monitor the patient closely in case she develops optic neuropathy as she may then need a lateral orbitotomy. The diagnosis is ... ?

81.   Which of the above lesions is similar to the one described in question 80 but has a more aggressive course, and tends to recur locally and metastasize?

Theme: Orbital lesions II

Options
A   Orbital varices
B   AV malformation
C   Lymphoma
D   Fibrous histiocytoma
E   Neurofibroma
F   Optic nerve glioma

For each of the clinical scenarios below, select the single most likely diagnosis from the list above. Each option may be used once, more than once or not at all.

82.   A 10-year-old child with Lisch nodules on the iris. She has a mass in the anterior orbit with thickening of the periorbital tissues. She has ...?

83.   A 57-year-old female patient presents in casualty. She has a deep purple mass visible superonasally in the anterior orbit. When she bends forward this is enlarging and the eyelid closes completely. The diagnosis is ...?

84.   A 60-year-old patient presents with a 4-week history of redness and chemosis of the right eye. There is a corkscrew pattern of the conjunctival vessels and the intraocular pressure is 24 mmHg in the right eye and 18 mmHg in the left eye. She has moderately controlled hypertension. MRI of the orbits and head shows an enlarged superior ophthalmic vein. You decide to order an orbital Doppler. You suspect ...?

Theme: Orbital lesions III

Options
A   Lymphangioma
B   Optic nerve glioma
C   Meningioma
D   Schwannoma
E   Rhabdomyosarcoma
F   Metastatic neuroblastoma

For each of the clinical scenarios below, select the single most likely diagnosis from the list above. Each option may be used once, more than once or not at all.

85. A 10-year-old girl presents with sudden onset of axial proptosis, loss of vision, RAPD and optic nerve swelling. An initial CT scan shows fusiform enlargement of the optic nerve. There is also a malformation of part of the sphenoid bone. The most likely diagnosis is . . . ?

86. A 55-year-old female patient has presented with axial proptosis, which has been gradually deteriorating for the past 4 months. There is chemosis and lid oedema, which are of recent onset. There is fullness of the temporal fossa. CT scan shows hyperostosis of the sphenoid bone and an associated soft tissue mass. The most likely diagnosis based on the history and CT scan findings is . . . ?

87. An 8-year-old child presents with sudden onset of proptosis and is admitted as an emergency. There is a palpable superonasal mass. CT scan shows a well-defined homogenous mass. T2-weighted MRI sequence shows that the mass is hyperintense to muscle and fat. You refer the child for a biopsy and the pathologist reports that it is an alveolar form of . . . ?

Theme: Orbit

Options
A Thyroid eye disease
B Orbital myositis
C Idiopathic orbital inflammatory disease
D Orbital apex syndrome
E Wegener's granulomatosis
F Orbital abscess

For each of the clinical scenarios below, select the single most likely diagnosis from the list above. Each option may be used once, more than once or not at all.

88. A 51-year-old lady has been referred by her GP to the anterior segment clinic because of recurrent eyelid swelling. On examination she has eyelid erythema and oedema and marked bilateral conjunctival chemosis. She has been suffering with this for the past 6 months. Ocular examination is unremarkable otherwise. You decide to investigate. What is the first condition you need to exclude?

89. A 29-year-old woman attends her clinic follow-up appointment. She has restriction of adduction in the left eye. Looking back through her notes, she was initially seen in the eye casualty 6 months ago complaining of sudden onset of orbital pain which was worse when adducting the left eye. She was treated with oral NSAIDs to which she responded well. She had a CT scan which was pathognomonic for her condition. She had a similar episode about a year ago in the same eye. Her eyes are healthy otherwise. The diagnosis is . . . ?

90. A 62-year-old man is seen in the eye casualty. Over the past 24 hours he has developed periorbital pain, diplopia and progressive proptosis. He has complete oculomotor paresis and numbness across his forehead. This is an emergency as it is a case of . . . ?

Theme: Management of orbital disease

Options
A   Monitor with VA testing, visual fields, clinical examination daily
B   Refer urgently to tertiary orbital centre for decompression
C   Refer for low dose orbital radiotherapy
D   Refer routinely to orbital specialist for orbital decompression
E   Consider immunosuppression
F   Immunosuppression and urgent radiotherapy

For each of the clinical scenarios below, select the single most likely treatment from the list above. Each option may be used once, more than once or not at all.

91.   A 43-year-old lady with TED has been stable for over 9 months now. The inflammation is inactive. She is off the oral steroids now. She has proptosis 24 mm in the right eye and 25 mm in the left eye. Intraocular pressures are 22 mmHg in the right eye and 26 mmHg in the left eye. She is concerned about her exophthalmos. What can you offer to her?

92.   A 46-year old male patient who also smokes about 20 cigarettes daily has been diagnosed with acute TED. He has significant inflammation and optic neuropathy. He has responded well to IV steroids and is now tapering off the oral steroids. His current daily dose is 20 mg. What is the next step in his management?

93.   You are treating a 63-year-old non-insulin-dependent diabetic man for acute TED with optic neuropathy. His visual acuity in the left eye has deteriorated from 6/9 to 6/36. The other eye is amblyopic. He has had the appropriate dose of systemic steroids, but the inflammation is not improving. You need to make a quick decision regarding his further management. What would be the most appropriate decision?

Theme: Treating orbital lesions

Options
A   Treat with IV methylprednisolone
B   Refer for radiotherapy
C   Treat with oral prednisolone and then refer to orbital specialist
D   Refer to orbital specialist for biopsy
E   Perform an urgent lateral canthotomy
F   Commence oral antibiotics

For each of the clinical scenarios below, select the single most likely treatment from the list above. Each option may be used once, more than once or not at all.

94. A patient has severe ocular pain when moving the eyes, especially at abduction of the left eye. She is not improving on oral NSAIDs. Her CT scan shows diffuse enlargement of the left lateral rectus muscle. The muscle tendon is involved as well. What is the next step in her treatment?

95. After investigating a patient thoroughly, you feel he may have an infiltrative orbital lesion. What do you decide to do now?

96. You are in the eye casualty at midnight and a 41-year-old gentleman is brought by the paramedics. He has been punched and kicked in the left eye. By the time you examine him his visual acuity has deteriorated, his orbit feels tense, there is massive chemosis, his intraocular pressure is raised and his eye movements are severely restricted. The globe is intact but you suspect a retrobulbar haemorrhage. What do you do?

Theme: Lacrimal gland

Options
A   Dacryoadenitits
B   Lymphoma
C   Pleomorphic adenoma of the lacrimal gland
D   Sarcoidosis
E   Idiopathic lacrimal gland inflammation
F   Dacryops

For each of the clinical scenarios below, select the single most likely diagnosis from the list above. Each option may be used once, more than once or not at all.

97.   A 50-year-old patient presents with painless, gradually progressing proptosis. Examination on slit lamp shows a subconjunctival mass superonasally. The mass has a 'salmon-patch' appearance. What is the possible diagnosis?

98.   A 61-year-old Afro-Carribean gentleman presents with a 4-week history of progressive downward and inward globe displacement. He complains of strong pain associated with it. It is progressive and unilateral. ACE and chest X-ray are normal. The CT scan shows a round well-circumscribed mass that is pressing the globe. There is no bony erosion. What is the most likely diagnosis?

99.   A 23-year-old man presents in the eye casualty. For the past month he has noticed a small cyst in the superotemporal area of his left eye. The cyst is not painful and its size is variable according to the history. He mentions that his eye starts to water suddenly. You examine the upper fornix and there is a large cyst. The diagnosis is . . . ?

Theme: Management of corneal exposure

Options
A   Lubricants and consider temporary tarsorraphy
B   Gold weight
C   Lateral canthal sling +/– medial canthoplasty
D   Lateral canthal sling +/– medial wedge resection
E   Lester Jones tube
F   Direct brow lift

For each of the clinical scenarios below, select the single most likely management from the list above. Each option may be used once, more than once or not at all.

100.   A 76-year-old patient had a VII nerve palsy 4 weeks ago. When you examine her she has a painful red eye. There is significant corneal exposure and she still can't shut her eye. She has a poor Bell's phenomenon. What is the appropriate management of this patient?

101.   You see the same patient 6 months later. Her condition has improved but the main problem seems to be the paralytic lower lid ectropion on the affected side. The medial canthal tendon is very lax. What surgical procedure would you consider?

102.   A patient comes for her follow-up. Her notes are missing. Only by observing her upper eyelid you understand she had facial nerve palsy in the past. What surgery did she have?

Theme: Corneal exposure

Options

A   Botulinum toxin injection to levator
B   Skin graft or Z-plasty
C   Recession of upper lid retractors +/– spacer
D   Decompression
E   Release of conjunctiva + MMG
F   Lateral tarsorraphy

For each of the clinical scenarios below, select the single most likely treatment from the list above. Each option may be used once, more than once or not at all.

103.   You are following up an inpatient in the eye ward. He is a 93-year-old disabled gentleman with a large sterile corneal ulcer at risk of perforation. He has an anaesthetic cornea. He is on quite a significant amount of topical medication which is starting to cause problems with corneal toxicity as well. He does not tolerate the bandage contact lens you inserted 2 days ago. The corneal epithelium does not appear to be healing any further. What option are you thinking about?

104.   A young patient has extensive scarring of the anterior lamella of his lower eyelid following an injury during which he sustained extensive lacerations in his face and eyelid that were repaired in a general hospital. He has problems with corneal exposure. What is the procedure that would offer him the best cosmetic and functional outcome?

105.   A patient asks for a second opinion. She had ptosis correction combined with upper lid blepharoplasty in another eye unit 9 months ago. She has been overcorrected and that has been managed conservatively by the other department. However her condition has not improved and she is now experiencing problems due to corneal exposure. She would like to consider another operation. What would be indicated in her case?

Theme: Congenital orbital malformations

Options
A   Crouzon's syndrome
B   Treacher Collins syndrome
C   Goldenhar's syndrome
D   Apert's syndrome
E   Hypertelorism
F   Microphthalmos

For each of the clinical scenarios below, select the single most likely diagnosis from the list above. Each option may be used once, more than once or not at all.

106.   You examine a 9-year-old girl who has a very wide mouth, hypoplastic maxilla and mandible on the right side, and a pre-auricular skin tag. She is wearing a hearing aid. She has a very small globe on the right side and an epibulbar dermoid encroaching on the right cornea. What is the diagnosis?

107.   A young boy attends with his mother. They both have abnormal facial characteristics. The mandible and zygoma in the boy's case are hypoplastic. His lateral canthus is lower than the medial canthus. They have . . . ?

108.   You are asked to examine a 3-year-old child, as there is concern about her cornea on the right side. Her orbits are very shallow which gives the impression of severe bilateral proptosis. There is a large distance between the two eyes and she has a marked exotropia especially on upgaze. Her optic discs look slightly pale.
       She most likely suffers with . . . ?

Theme: Socket

Options
A   Post-enucleation socket syndrome
B   Elephant syndrome
C   Contracted socket
D   Ocular surface breakdown
E   Extrusion of implant
F   Chronic socket infection

For each of the clinical scenarios below, select the single most likely diagnosis from the list above. Each option may be used once, more than once or not at all.

109.   A patient with prosthesis has been referred by his GP to have surgical correction of his lower eyelid that has become droopy on the side of the prosthesis. On examination the prosthesis is displaced downward and appears to be unstable and the lower lid has become very lax. There is almost no inferior fornix. This is called ...?

110.   A patient with an artificial eye attends his clinic follow-up. He tells you that in the past 2 years he has had two new larger prostheses fitted. Despite that he still feels that the eye with the prosthesis 'doesn't look right'. On examination he has enophthalmos, the upper sulcus is very deep and the upper eyelid is ptotic. The problem is ...?

111.   A child with prosthesis. The mother has noticed problems in the past 6 months. On examination the fornices are very shallow and there is conjunctival scarring. There is entropion of the lower lid and the prosthesis looks particularly unstable. What is the name of the socket problem in this case?

Theme: Orbital trauma

Options
A   Observation
B   Repair within 24–48 hours
C   Repair within 2 weeks
D   Repair within 1 week
E   Surgical repair not necessary
F   Refer to neurosurgery

For each of the clinical scenarios below, select the single most likely management from the list above. Each option may be used once, more than once or not at all.

112.   You are asked to examine a child following a RTA. The child is unwell and has an orbital floor fracture, which is obvious on the CT scan. There is a definite entrapment of the inferior rectus muscle in the fracture. What is the appropriate management?

113.   A young man has been involved in a fight and hit in the face with a blunt heavy instrument. He has multiple fractures of the nose and sinuses. He is complaining of horizontal diplopia and he has enophthalmos. CT scan shows a medial orbital wall fracture with medial rectus entrapment. What do you advise?

114.   A 25-year-old man has an orbital roof fracture confirmed on CT. What is the appropriate course of action?

Chapter 2

Cornea and External Eye Disease – EMQs

- This chapter consists of 66 extended matching questions.
- Questions consist of a theme, a list of options, an instruction and a variable number of clinical situations.
- For each of the clinical situations, you should choose the **single most likely option** according to the instruction.
- It is possible for one option to be the answer to more than one of the clinical situations.

Chapter 2: Cornea and External Eye Disease EMQs

Theme: Ectasias

Options
A   Keratoconus
B   Pellucid marginal degeneration
C   Keratoglobus
D   Posterior keratoconus
E   Cornea plana
F   Keractasia

For each of the clinical scenarios below, select the single most likely diagnosis from the list above. Each option may be used once, more than once or not at all.

1.   A young man married to his cousin presents to external disease clinic. He gives a history of sudden onset unilateral blurring of vision following a history of minimal trauma. On systemic enquiry you discover a history of multiple bone fractures and difficulty in hearing. On general examination he has hyperextensible joints. On slit-lamp examination you observe bilateral corneal thinning out to the periphery with associated scleral thinning. There is paracentral scarring and intrastromal clefts as seen in hydrops.

2.   A young patient presents with bilateral progressive blurring of vision. His optician's report reveals marked irregular astigmatism that is now difficult to correct with spectacles. On slit-lamp examination you see bilateral corneal thinning 1–2 mm in width, extending from 4 o'clock to 8 o'clock inferiorly An area of normal corneal thickness protrudes above the area of thinning and looks like a 'beer belly'. Orbscan shows superior against-the-rule astigmatism and inferior with-the-rule astigmatism.

3.   A baby with Peter's anomaly also has bilateral reduction in corneal curvature, shallow anterior chambers and glaucoma. Refraction reveals marked hypermetropia.

Theme: Conjunctival disorders

Options
A   Ocular cicatricial pemphigoid
B   Erythema multiforme major
C   Kaposi's sarcoma
D   Conjunctival lymphoma
E   Ligneous conjunctivitis
F   Trachoma

For each of the clinical scenarios below, select the single most likely diagnosis from the list above. Each option may be used once, more than once or not at all.

4. A small elderly Pakistani lady attends your clinic complaining of bilateral sore eyes and foreign body sensation. On examination of her anterior segment you see Arlt's line on everting both lids, Herbert's pits at the limbus, bilateral scarring of both corneas. There is no evidence of active inflammation.

5. A young man of 28 presents with acute, self-limited, non-progressive, inflammatory disorders of the skin and mucous membranes, following malaise, fever and headache, mouth ulcers, bilateral red eyes, mucopurulent discharge at 4 weeks. He now has bilateral symblepharon, entropion, trichiasis and the cornea is vascularized and opacified.

6. A 70-year-old man presents with chronic unilateral red eye. On examination there is a single raised, oval, 'salmon' patch on the temporal bulbar conjunctiva. It is painless.

Theme: Acute conjunctivitis

Options
A   Gonococcal
B   Adenoviral serotype 8
C   Adenoviral serotype 3
D   Chlamydial
E   HSV-1
F   Allergic

For each of the clinical scenarios below, select the single most likely diagnosis from the list above. Each option may be used once, more than once or not at all.

7.   A young man attends casualty with a 2-day history of severely purulent discharge and lid swelling in his right eye. He has conjunctival papillae, chemosis and pre-auricular lymphadenopathy. There is no corneal ulcer. A conjunctival swab is sent off for urgent Gram stain. He is treated with topical and systemic antibiotics and referred to GU clinic.

8.   A young woman attends casualty with bilateral asymmetrical red eyes. She is pyrexial, complains of malaise and a sore throat. On examination she has pre-auricular and mandibular lymphadenopathy, conjunctival follicles, bulbar conjunctival injection. Her partner has a similar complaint.

9.   A young atopic woman who has just returned from a skiing holiday complains of bilateral red, sore eyes associated with a foreign body sensation. She has vesicles around the lids and staining on the cornea.

Theme: Chronic conjunctivitis

Options
A   Molluscum
B   Atopic
C   Trachoma
D   Staphylococcal
E   Rosacea
F   Graft-versus-host disease

For each of the clinical scenarios below, select the single most likely diagnosis from the list above. Each option may be used once, more than once or not at all.

10.   A middle-aged man has been attending the external disease clinic for years. On examination he has facial hyperaemia, lid margin telangiectasia, bilateral trichiasis, posterior dragging of the grey line, sebhorroeic blepharoconjunctivitis, pannus and peripheral corneal thinning.

11.   An HIV-positive young man complains of recurrent history of right red eye for the past 2 years. He describes periods of remission and exacerbation. On examination he has a papillary reaction and in between the lashes there are small nodules, which have been missed on previous examination. These nodules are treated by cryotherapy.

12.   An elderly Asian woman from Kenya has bilateral trichiasis, scarring of tarsal conjunctiva, scarred limbal follicles, marked corneal scarring. She is due to have punctual cautery for her evaporative dry eyes.

Theme: Cicatrizing conjunctivitis

Options
A Linear IgA disease
B Ocular cicatricial pemphigoid
C Erythema multiforme
D Toxic epidermal necrolysis
E Adenoviral conjunctivitis
F Alkali injury

For each of the clinical scenarios below, select the single most likely diagnosis from the list above. Each option may be used once, more than once or not at all.

13. A 45-year-old man overweight from long-term systemic steroid use enters the clinic. He has a history of multiple lid procedures, bilateral large symblepharon, corneal vascularization, oral mucosal ulcers, and desquammative gingivitis has damaged his teeth. Vancomycin has been implicated as the causative agent.

14. An elderly woman has been attending the cornea clinic for 10 years. She has a keratoprosthesis in her right eye. The left eye is mildly injected, she has marked corneal vascularization and scarring, ankyloblepharon, shortened fornices, obliteration of meibomian gland ducts. She is on frequent preservative-free ocular lubricants and systemic oral prednisolone and dapsone.

15. An 18-year-old woman was treated 1 week ago with trimethoprim-sulfamethoxazole for a urinary tract infection. She complains of a 3-day history of blistering over her entire body. There is also inflammation of her mucosal tissue lips, throat, labia and conjunctival mucosa. She has a rash on her body and bilateral red eyes following a course of penicillin. She required admission to a burns unit to prevent sloughing of further tissue and supportive measures included intravenous fluids. She stabilized over 3 weeks.

Theme: Herpes simplex virus

Options
A   Endotheliitis
B   Stromal keratitis
C   Neurotrophic keratopathy
D   HEDS II
E   Acute retinal necrosis
F   HEDS I

For each of the statements below, select the single most likely option from the list above. Each option may be used once, more than once or not at all.

16.   A patient with known HSV keratitis presents to casualty with an acute red eye. He has stromal oedema without stromal infiltrates. He also has keratic precipitates and iritis. His intraocular pressure is normal. There are no posterior segment findings.

17.   A patient with a history of frequent recurrent HSV keratitis presents to casualty with a red eye. Her vision is 6/60. The epithelium is intact. There are multiple punctate stromal opacities accompanied by haze. There is a mild AC reaction and associated discomfort.

18.   This study showed that patients with epithelial keratitis are best treated with topical antiviral therapy and oral acyclovir does not provide any additional benefit. Patients with stromal keratitis treated with oral acyclovir for 12 months had a 50% reduction in the rate of recurrent stromal keratitis.

Theme: Interstitial keratitis

Options
A   Onchocerciasis
B   Congenital syphilis
C   Leprosy
D   Cogan's syndrome
E   Epstein–Barr virus
F   Sarcoidosis

For each of the clinical scenarios below, select the single most likely diagnosis from the list above. Each option may be used once, more than once or not at all.

19.   A middle-aged man presents with rapid onset ocular pain, watering and photophobia. On examination there is iritis, subconjunctival haemorrhage, patchy anterior-stromal opacification. A few weeks later he developed nausea, vomiting, tinnitus, vertigo and hearing loss. Further investigation by a physician revealed an underlying granulomatous systemic condition.

20.   A young man from East Africa presents to casualty with intense conjunctivitis and pruritis. Around his eyelids he has marked scarring that has a 'leopard skin' appearance. He also has painless dermal nodules on his forehead. On slit-lamp examination he has stromal opacities, granulomatous keratic precipitates. Posterior segment examination reveals RPE atrophy and chorioretinal atrophy.

21.   A 35-year-old Afro-Caribbean woman attends clinic. She has bilateral hilar lymphadenopathy on chest X-ray.

Theme: Therapeutic indications for contact lens wear

Options

A   Thygeson's keratitis
B   Superior limbic keratoconjunctivitis
C   Bullous keratopathy
D   Aphakia
E   Exposure keratopathy
F   Recurrent erosion

For each of the clinical scenarios below, select the single most likely diagnosis from the list above. Each option may be used once, more than once or not at all.

22.   A patient attends clinic complaining of foreign body sensation, pain and mucoid discharge. On examination there is conjunctival hyperaemia and fine papillae. Superior bulbar and limbal conjunctiva shows sectoral injection and is thickened and redundant. There is a superior punctate epithelial keratitis. Rose Bengal shows coarse punctate staining of the superior bulbar conjunctiva. There are superior corneal filaments that require removal and topical acetyl-cysteine.

23.   A 25-year-old woman was scratched in her eye by her baby 18 months ago. Since then she has attended casualty at 1- to 2-month intervals complaining of pain and photophobia. She has bilateral corneal epithelial defects obvious on fluorescein staining.

24.   A 20-year-old attends contact lens clinic. She had bilateral congenital cataracts removed as a baby and now wears rigid gas permeable contact lenses.

Theme: Complications of contact lens wear

Options
A   Giant papillary conjunctivitis
B   Sterile infiltrates
C   Hypoxia
D   Acanthamoeba keratitis
E   Dessication
F   Microtrauma

For each of the clinical scenarios below, select the single most likely diagnosis from the list above. Each option may be used once, more than once or not at all.

25.   A patient attends casualty with sore eyes. He wears daily-wear soft contact lenses for about 16 hours a day. On examination there are epithelial microcysts, corneal oedema and 360 degrees superficial vascularization.

26.   A woman presents to casualty with mildly painful red eye for a few days. On examination there are multiple subepithelial infiltrates. There is no overlying staining with fluorescein. The anterior chamber is quiet.

27.   A 30-year-old man wears extended-wear soft contact lenses. On examination he has macropapillae up to 1 mm in diameter. He uses topical mast cell stabilizer and keeps his daily wear time to a minimum.

Theme: Secondary causes of corneal astigmatism

Options
A   Pellucid marginal degeneration
B   Terrien's marginal degeneration
C   Mooren's ulcer
D   Post-infectious scar
E   Keratoconus
F   None of the above

For each of the clinical scenarios below, select the single most likely diagnosis from the list above. Each option may be used once, more than once or not at all.

28.   A 20-year-old man with Marfan's syndrome is reviewed in contact lens clinic. Signs on slit-lamp examination include Fleischer's ring, Rizutti's sign, Munson's sign and paracentral stromal thinning. Retinoscopy reveals a scissor reflex.

29.   This is a rare condition, seen in men in 75% of cases. Occurs in over-40s. It is a slowly progressive bilateral condition. The peripheral thinning starts in the superior cornea and progresses circumferentially. It is usually steep centrally and shallow peripherally. Superficial radial vessels fill the gutter and deposit lipid. It is rarely painful.

30.   This is an idiopathic peripheral macroulcerative keratitis. The rapidly progressive inflammatory type is seen in younger patients associated with painful episodes of episcleritis and scleritis. In older patients the condition is slowly progressive and asymptomatic for long periods. It is a diagnosis of exclusion following systemic investigations that are negative for vasculitis and connective tissue disorders. An ulcer is classically described as an aggressive peripheral ulceration with a steep, deeply undermined and infiltrated central edge. It progresses centrally and circumferentially.

Theme: Corneal graft surgery

Options

A   Penetrating keratoplasty
B   Tectonic keratoplasty
C   Deep lamellar endothelial keratoplasty
D   Deep anterior lamellar keratoplasty
E   Keratoprosthesis
F   Large diameter penetrating keratoplasty

For each of the clinical scenarios below, select the single most likely treatment from the list above. Each option may be used once, more than once or not at all.

31.   A 60-year-old woman complains of blurry vision in the mornings that improves somewhat during the course of the day. On pachymetry her central corneal thickness is 650 µm and peripheral 600 µm. There are central and peripheral guttata, stromal oedema and epithelial oedema. Which of the above surgical techniques would be ideal?

32.   A 45-year-old man has unilateral corneal pannus, anterior to mid stromal vascularization, scarring and lipid deposition. He describes a past history of recurrent conjunctivitis. Looking through his notes there is no history of uveitis or endotheliitis. He has a history of cold sores on his lips. Which of the above surgical techniques would be ideal?

33.   A 30-year-old referred by his optician has high against-the-rule astigmatism and peripheral corneal changes. On examination there is 20% thinning of the peripheral cornea at the limbus between the 4 and 8 o'clock positions. There is no vascularization. There is no scarring. There are endothelial stress lines and hydrops. Spectacles and contact lenses improve his vision very little. Which of the above surgical techniques would be ideal?

Theme: Corneal opacity and scarring

Options
A   Trachoma
B   Disciform keratitis
C   Band keratopathy
D   Interstitial keratitis
E   Verticillata
F   None of the above

For each of the clinical scenarios below, select the single most likely diagnosis from the list above. Each option may be used once, more than once or not at all.

34.   A 19-year-old is followed up several times a year in the uveitis clinic. She has pauciarticular juvenile chronic arthritis. She is ANA positive and has chronic anterior uveitis in both eyes. There are corneal opacities in both eyes in the interpalpebral region.

35.   Cardiologists refer a patient on amiodarone 50 mg once-daily. What would you expect to see on slit-lamp examination of this patient's cornea?

36.   This condition is a manifestation of both non-infectious and infectious diseases. On examination you see cellular infiltration and vascularization. There is minimal involvement of the corneal epithelium and endothelium. It can be caused by direct invasion of the cornea by microorganisms or by immune response against foreign antigen.

Theme: Corneal disease associated with systemic diseases

Options
A   Rheumatoid arthritis
B   Systemic lupus erythematosus
C   Systemic sclerosis
D   Wegener's granulomatosis
E   Polyarteritis nodosa
F   Churg–Strauss syndrome

For each of the clinical scenarios below, select the single most likely diagnosis from the list above. Each option may be used once, more than once or not at all.

37.   Allergic symptoms including asthma for many years followed by eosinophilia in blood and tissues, followed by vasculitis. It is common in males with an onset around 40 years. Aetiology is unknown. Histology shows necrotizing vasculitis of small arteries and veins. This is a very rare condition and ocular problems have been infrequently reported, eg episcleritis, scleritis, conjunctival nodular thickening and uveitis.

38.   A systemic vasculitic disorder characterized by necrotizing and granulomatous inflammation of the vessels of the upper respiratory tract, glomerulonephritis and other organs with small vessels. Onset is in the mid-40s. Male : female = 2 : 1. Patients complain of fever, malaise, arthralgia, sinusitis, epistaxis. Ocular inflammation is seen in over 50%. Ocular finding include proptosis from an orbital lesion, nasolacrimal duct obstruction, ischaemic optic neuropathy, retinal artery or vein occlusion. Anterior segment findings include episcleritis, non-necrotizing and necrotizing scleritis, keratitis involving subepithelial opacities and peripheral ulcerative keratitis.

39.   A mulitsytsem disorder causing fibrosis of skin and viscera. Vast majority of patients are women. In CREST (Calcinosis, Raynaud's, (o)Esophagitis, Sclerodactyly, Telangiectasia) syndrome visceral involvement is less common. Ocular manifestations are common: eyelid tightening. blepharophimosis, exposure keratopathy, shallowing of conjunctival fornices, keratoconjunctivitis sicca. Orbital findings are rare.

Theme: Corneal dystrophies

Options
A   Meesman's dystrophy
B   Reis–Buckler dystrophy
C   Granular dystrophy
D   Macular dystrophy
E   Avellino dystrophy
F   Schnyder's crystalline dystrophy

For each of the clinical scenarios below, select the single most likely dystrophy from the list above. Each option may be used once, more than once or not at all.

40.   This dystrophy has an autosomal recessive inheritance. Of the three classic stromal dystrophies this is the least common and the most severe. Patients complain of irritation and progressive loss of vision by their 20s or 30s. The opacification is characterized by diffuse, cloudy opacities of the central stroma with no clear intervening spaces. As it progresses it extends to the periphery and involves the entire thickness of the cornea when advanced. Corneal thickness is reduced.

41.   This is a variant of granular dystrophy in which there are lattice deposits. Patients experience foreign body sensation, pain and photophobia secondary to recurrent erosions. Recurrent granular deposits have been noted on donor grafts.

42.   This is an epithelial basement membrane dystrophy. Patients have characteristic changes in the corneal epithelium: microcystic, map-like patterns, fingerprint-like lines, more unusually bleb-like changes are seen. Patients complain of pain due to recurrent erosions. These can be treated by anterior stromal puncture or phototherapeutic keratectomy.

Theme: Ocular causes of peripheral ulcerative keratitis

Options
A   Pellucid marginal degeneration
B   Marginal keratitis
C   Terrien's marginal degeneration
D   Mooren's
E   Acne rosacea
F   Neurotrophic keratopathy

For each of the clinical scenarios below, select the single most likely diagnosis from the list above. Each option may be used once, more than once or not at all.

43.   A 45-year-old woman has persistent erythematous papules, pustules and hypertrophy of sebaceous glands on her face. She has bilateral blepharitis and multiple chalazions, there are papillary changes on tarsal conjunctiva. On her cornea there are punctate epithelial keratitis, subepithelial opacifications, peripheral thinning and vascularization.

44.   A patient is referred by her GP with a right red eye. She has had a resection of a right acoustic neuroma. There is a reduced blink reflex. The tear film is viscous because of increased mucous secretions. There is an epithelial defect with raised edges. Despite adequate lubrication, stromal lysis has ensued and resulted in peripheral thinning that could be at risk of perforating.

45.   A patient has bilateral staphylococcal blepharitis and has attended casualty on multiple occasions over the past 2 years with a red eye and requiring topical steroid treatment. She now has peripheral thinning at sites of previous infiltration.

Theme: Systemic causes of peripheral ulcerative keratitis

Options
A   Rheumatoid arthritis
B   Systemic lupus erythematosus
C   Sarcoidosis
D   Polyarteritis nodosa
E   Relapsing polychondritis
F   Leukaemia

For each of the clinical scenarios below, select the single most likely cause from the list above. Each option may be used once, more than once or not at all.

46.   A disorder of unknown aetiology more frequent in women (female:male = 9:1). It is a multisystem disorder. Characterized by malar rash, oral ulcers, non-erosive arthritis, pleuritis/pericarditis, glomerulonephritis, seizures, psychosis, haematological disorders such as haemolytic anaemia, lymphopenia or thrombocytopenia.

47.   A non-caseating granulomatous condition. Usually presents in young adults. Patients can present with bilateral hilar lymphadenopathy and erythema nodosum. Acute presentation can involve parotid gland enlargement. Ocular features include lupus pernio, anterior or panuveitis, retinitis, choroidal granulomas and optic nerve infiltration.

48.   This condition is diagnosed if three or more of the following are present: recurrent chondritis of auricles, arteritis, non-erosive inflammatory polyarthritis, chondritis of nasal cartilages, ocular inflammation, chondritis of tracheal/largyngeal cartilage, cochlear or vestibular damage causing tinnitus or vertigo. About 50% of patients have ocular manifestations: orbital inflammation, lid oedema, extraocular muscle palsy, conjunctival oedema, scleritis, uveitis and keratitis.

Theme: Microbial keratitis

Options
A   Fungal keratitis
B   Acanthamoeba keratitis
C   Pseudomonas keratitis
D   HSV keratitis
E   HZV keratitis
F   Gonococcal keratitis

For each of the clinical scenarios below, select the single most likely diagnosis from the list above. Each option may be used once, more than once or not at all.

49.   This keratitis caused by Gram-negative diplococci can present as a suppurative conjunctivitis. The bacteria invade into the epithelial cells via cell surface proteins and integrins causing phagocytosis. The bacteria proliferate within the corneal stroma and release proteolytic enzymes that destroy the stromal matrices and collagen fibrils. This needs to be treated promptly to avoid perforation.

50.   This vision-threatening infection is caused by an organism which in its dormant form exists as cysts and in its active form as tropho-zoites. Infection occurs in immunocompetent hosts who are contact lens wearers, have been exposed to contaminated water or contact lens solution. Patients typically present with severe pain out of proportion to clinical signs. Epithelial irregularity is a sign of early infection. Later on infection will present as single or multiple dense white stromal opacities and characteristically a ring stromal infiltrate. Radial keratoneuritis is present in fewer patients.

51.   This is the most common Gram-negative pathogen isolated from severe keratitis in the UK. In developed countries this is largely associated with soft contact lens wear. Characteristic findings include rapid progression, dense stromal infiltrate, marked suppuration, liquefactive necrosis, descemetocoele formation and corneal perforation. Progression can occur despite appropriate treatment.

Theme: Treatment options

Options
A   Oral tetracycline
B   Topical erythromycin ointment
C   Topical acetylcysteine drops
D   Topical mast cell stabilizer drops
E   Topical biguanide and diamidine drops
F   Topical intensive steroid drops

For each of the clinical scenarios below, select the single most likely treatment from the list above. Each option may be used once, more than once or not at all.

52.   This infection is seen in patients who are contact lens wearers. It is caused by a free-living protozoa. Symptoms are out of proportion with the signs. Textbook signs are stromal ring infiltrates and radial keratoneuritis. Which of the above is the most appropriate treatment?

53.   Bilateral collarettes and oily crusting of lid margins, erythema, lash misdirection is treated with daily lid hygiene. Which of the above is a useful treatment?

54.   A 10-year-old boy has eczema and hayfever. He complains of bilateral ocular pruritis, redness and chemosis. On eversion he has bilateral tarsal papillae. What would you use to treat this?

Theme: Systemic treatment options

Options
A   Dapsone
B   Cyclophosphamide
C   Azathioprine
D   Mycophenolate
E   Prednisolone
F   None of the above

For each of the clinical scenarios below, select the single most suitable systemic treatment from the list above. Each option may be used once, more than once or not at all.

55.   A patient is referred to the cornea clinic. She is 55 years old and has bilateral mild redness and dry, gritty sensation in both eyes that has been present for some months now. On examination there is mild conjunctival injection, inferior fornix symblepharon, subepithelial fibrosis and forniceal shortening, marked meibomianitis and trichiasis.

56.   A young man with epistaxis and a history of sinusitis presents with an injected, tender, left eye. B-scan shows thickening of posterior scleral coats. He known to be c-ANCA positive and is on systemic prednisolone already.

57.   A woman of 40 years of age has rheumatoid arthritis. She presents to casualty with a red right eye and peripheral ulcerative keratitis and anterior scleritis. There is 80% corneal thinning in the periphery. Conjunctival swabs and corneal scrapes are taken to exclude an infectious cause. She is given topical lubricants and requires urgent systemic treatment.

Theme: How would you manage this?

Options
A PTK
B Anterior stromal puncture
C Tectonic corneal graft
D Cauterization
E EDTA
F Scrape off a sheet of corneal epithelial cells for culture

For each of the clinical scenarios below, select the single most likely management option from the list above. Each option may be used once, more than once or not at all.

58. A 30-year-old myope has had multiple retinal detachments in one eye and has silicone oil in that eye. As a result he has deposition of calcium in Bowman's membrane. It fills the entire interpalpebral region and is affecting his vision. How would you remove this?

59. A man suffered a minor trauma to his corneal epithelium from the edge of a piece of paper a few years ago. Since then he wakes up in the morning with excruciating pain. He uses frequent lubricants and has tried bandage contact lenses but the area of epithelial defect soon breaks down again. What would you try first from the above?

60. A soft contact lens wearer presents to casualty with a ring infiltrate and radial perineural infiltrates and an excruciatingly painful eye. How should you manage this?

Theme: Prominent corneal nerves

Options
A   Keratoconus
B   Congenital glaucoma
C   Refsum's disease
D   Leprosy
E   Neurofibromatosis type 1
F   Multiple endocrine neoplasia type IIb

For each of the clinical scenarios below, select the single most likely diagnosis from the list above. Each option may be used once, more than once or not at all.

61. This is a retinitis pigmentosa with systemic associations consisting of phytanic acid metabolic abnormality, peripheral neuropathy, cardiac arrhythmias and cerebellar ataxia. Treatment involves phytanic acid free diet and plasma exchange.

62. This is a neurocutaneous syndrome. It has autosomal dominant inheritance with incomplete penetrance. Skin signs consist of café au lait spots, plexiform neurofibromas, tumours of the brain, spinal cord, cranial nerves and peripheral nerves. Orbital features include: proptosis due to optic nerve glioma or spheno-orbital encephalocoele, prominent corneal nerves, Lisch nodules on the iris, ectropian uvae, secondary glaucoma, choroidal hamartomas. Short stature, scoliosis, macrocephaly, facial hemiatrophy, phaeochromocytoma causing hypertension.

63. Patients can present with photophobia and epiphora. They may have axial myopia due to buphthalmos, enlarged vertical and horizontal corneal diameters, cloudy cornea, Haab's striae, cupped disc reversible with appropriate treatment.

Theme: Managing Fuch's endothelial dystrophy

Options

A   Observation
B   Triple procedure (cataract extraction, IOL implant and penetrating keratoplasty)
C   Cataract extraction alone
D   Cataract extraction and PK if cornea subsequently decompensates
E   Penetrating keratoplasty
F   Bandage contact lens

For each of the clinical scenarios below, select the single most suitable management option from the list above. Each option may be used once, more than once or not at all.

64.   A patient complains of misty vision when she wakes up in the mornings. During the day her eyes are sore. On examination she has a corneal thickness of 580 μm and a dense nuclear sclerotic cataract. Her vision is 6/36 unaided and improves to 6/18 with pinhole. Fundoscopy is unremarkable.

65.   A 65-year-old man has reduced vision, a cloudy cornea 575 μm in thickness, central and peripheral guttate, and an endothelial cell count of 600 cells/mm^2 and painful photophobic eyes when not wearing contact lenses. There is a cortical cataract.

66.   A 70-year-old woman has a corneal thickness of 545 μm on pachymetry and central corneal guttate. She has a nuclear sclerotic cataract and a visual acuity of 6/9 in that eye. She is asymptomatic.

Chapter 3

Refractive Surgery – EMQs

- This chapter consists of 12 extended matching questions.
- Questions consist of a theme, a list of options, an instruction and a variable number of clinical situations.
- For each of the clinical situations, you should choose the **single most likely option** according to the instruction.
- It is possible for one option to be the answer to more than one of the clinical situations.

Chapter 3: Refractive Surgery EMQs

Theme: Refractive procedures

Options

A   Radial keratotomy
B   Laser in situ keratomileusis (LASIK) for myopia
C   Epikeratoplasty
D   Laser in situ keratomileusis (LASIK) for hyperopia
E   Photorefractive keratectomy (PRK)
F   Laser-assisted subepithelial keratomileusis (LASEK)

For each of the clinical scenarios below, select the single most likely procedure from the list above. Each option may be used once, more than once or not at all.

1.   In this procedure donor corneal tissue is pre-lathed into shape and sutured onto recipient, de-epithelialized corneal tissue in which Bowman's layer and stroma have been left intact. This lenticule changes the curvature of the anterior surface and provides refractive correction.

2.   Microkeratome creates a corneal flap that is hinged. The flap is reflected. Excimer laser ablation remodels the cornea by removing stromal tissue. The flap is replaced. Which type of refractive error is corrected using this method that increases the central radius of curvature, making the cornea flatter with less optical power?

3.   In this procedure radial incisions of 85–95% corneal depth are made in the peripheral cornea with the aim of structurally weakening the cornea, which then allows the intraocular pressure and bio-mechanical forces to induce a change in its curvature.

Theme: LASIK complications

Options
A   Diffuse lamellar keratitis type 2
B   Epithelial ingrowth
C   Postoperative ectasia
D   Dislodged flap
E   Diffuse lamellar keratitis type 4
F   Flap striae type 3

For each of the clinical scenarios below, select the single most likely diagnosis from the list above. Each option may be used once, more than once or not at all.

4.   This complication occurs 1–7 days postoperatively. It is a postoperative interface inflammation. The incidence is 1 : 200 to 1 : 500 cases. It presents as diffuse, confluent, white to grey granular material under the flap. It is localized to a central 2–4 mm. There are central interface striae. The vision is markedly reduced and there is no anterior chamber reaction. Treatment involves interface irrigation, intensive topical steroids, topical antibiotics and close observation.

5.   Sometimes the flap rolls onto itself. In most cases this occurs within an hour after surgery. This can vary in severity – sometimes it can cause glare, haloes, diplopia. It can reduce vision to below 6/12 and is obvious on retro-illumination. There is >1 D astigmatism.

6.   A patient is reviewed for his postoperative visit. A faint grey line is seen extending 1 mm from the flap edge. Visual acuity is not reduced. He does however complain of a mild foreign body sensation.

Theme: Correcting hyperopia

Options
A   Thermal keratoplasty
B   Conductive keratoplasty
C   LASEK
D   Anterior chamber phakic IOL
E   PRK
F   LASIK

For each of the clinical scenarios below, select the single most likely procedure from the list above. Each option may be used once, more than once or not at all.

7. In this procedure corneal epithelium is loosened with alcohol and scrolled back to expose Bowman's layer. After excimer laser treatment the epithelium is replaced and a bandage contact lens is fitted.

8. This technique steepens the corneal curvature thus increasing its refractive power. It spares the central cornea and doesn't involve the removal of stromal tissue. A holmium : YAG laser system is used to create eight equidistant spots located circumferentially at a 6 mm zone followed by a second ring of spots at a 7 mm zone.

9. This procedure involves removal of corneal epithelium mechanically/by laser, followed by ablation of Bowman's layer. Bandage contact lens is required during re-epithelialization. Corrects up to −6 D.

Theme: Correcting myopia

Options

A   Scleral sling
B   Epikeratoplasty
C   Iris fixated phakic intraocular lens
D   Intrastromal corneal rings
E   Clear lens extraction and intraocular lens implantation
F   LASEK

For each of the clinical scenarios below, select the single most likely diagnosis from the list above. Each option may be used once, more than once or not at all.

10.   A 30-year-old patient wants to discuss reducing her –4 D of myopia. She has a history of atopy and bilateral HSV keratitis. She is intolerant to contact lenses and would like to discuss options in order to avoid wearing glasses.

11.   A patient with keratoconus has had a deep lamellar endothelial keratoplasty in one eye and is supposed to wear rigid gas permeable contact lenses in the other eye. He has become intolerant to his contact lens and is asking for options other than a corneal graft.

12.   A patient is being worked up for cataract extraction and tells you that many decades ago she had a procedure that involved 'changing the shape of her globe to make her eye longer'. She describes the use of a synthetic material. She has a preoperative B-scan.

Chapter 4

Glaucoma – EMQs

- This chapter consists of 30 extended matching questions.
- Questions consist of a theme, a list of options, an instruction and a variable number of clinical situations.
- For each of the clinical situations, you should choose the **single most likely option** according to the instruction.
- It is possible for one option to be the answer to more than one of the clinical situations.

Chapter 4: Glaucoma EMQs

Theme: Acute raised intraocular pressure

Options

A   Primary angle closure with pupil block
B   Angle closure without pupil block
C   Posner–Schlossman syndrome
D   Eight ball hyphaema
E   Schwartz syndrome
F   Aqueous misdirection

For each of the clinical scenarios below, select the single most likely diagnosis from the list above. Each option may be used once, more than once or not at all.

1. It is mid-November and an elderly woman attends casualty with a painful, red eye she has had for 2 days. She says her vision is blurry and she is feeling nauseated. You observe that she is wearing glasses that magnify both eyes. There is no past ocular history to note. On examination the pressure is 52 mmHg in the affected eye, her vision is reduced compared to the other eye. There is a cloudy cornea, activity in the anterior chamber, dilated irregular pupil, iris bombe, gonioscopy shows 360 degrees Schaffer grading 0–1. The disc is difficult to see but appears healthy.

2. A myopic man presents with an aching right eye. He has an IOP of 45 mmHg in that eye. Gonioscopy reveals an open angle with marked pigment deposition compared to none in the other eye. On examining his posterior segment he is Schaffer positive and has a large retinal detachment associated with multiple tears.

3. A 35-year-old woman complains of mild pain and haloes in her right eye. She has had this on and off for a few months now. On examination the intraocular pressure in that eye is 60 mmHg. There are a few fine keratic precipitates on the corneal endothelium. Gonioscopy reveals an open angle and no peripheral anterior synechiae. She is started on intensive topical steroids, medical treatment to reduce her intraocular pressure.

Theme: What is the cause of low intraocular pressure?

Options
A   Angle recession
B   Chronic anterior uveitis
C   Bleb leak
D   Excessive filtration from bleb
E   Overfiltration from drainage device
F   None of the above

For each of the clinical scenarios below, select the single most likely diagnosis from the list above. Each option may be used once, more than once or not at all.

4. A 21-year-old man attends casualty with reduction in vision over the course of the day. He is very anxious as his visual acuity RE is 6/60 unaided and 6/24 with pinhole. He has a history of chronic anterior uveitis and is HLA B27+ve. Seven days ago he had a right Baerveldt tube with supramid inserted into the lumen and scleral patch graft. On examination his intraocular pressure is 4 mmHg, The anterior chamber is shallow. The optic disc is swollen, there is macular oedema and choroidal folds. He requires viscoelastic injected into his anterior chamber.

5. A 30-year-old man presents to casualty following a blunt trauma to his left eye while playing squash. Facial X-rays are unremarkable. He has an intraocular pressure of 3 mmHg in his left eye. The anterior chamber has 2+ cells. The globe is intact. Gonioscopy shows the iris torn from its insertion into the ciliary body in the superior quadrant. There is no cataract. There is maculopathy. There are no choroidal folds and the disc is unaffected.

6. A patient is seen one day postop. following a fornix-based trabeculectomy with mitomycin C. On examination the intraocular pressure is 6 mmHg. The anterior chamber is deep. There is a Siedel's positive sign at the site of nasal limbal conjunctival sutures. There is no maculopathy, choroidal folds or disc swelling.

Theme: Secondary glaucomas

Options
A   Irido-corneal endothelial syndrome
B   Axenfeld–Rieger syndrome
C   Traumatic angle recession
D   Complete aniridia
E   Pigment dispersion syndrome
F   Pseudoexfoliative glaucoma

For each of the clinical scenarios below, select the single most likely diagnosis from the list above. Each option may be used once, more than once or not at all.

7. You are in clinic and follow up a Caucasian man who complains his eye aches after a session at the gym. You note that he is myopic. On examination you notice he has deep anterior chambers, pigment deposition on corneal endothelium and Schwalbe's line, mid-peripheral posterior bowing of the iris and lattice degeneration.

8. A middle-aged Cauacasian woman is followed up in clinic. Findings on examination are in one eye. You notice a Seton device, a penetrating keratoplasty, marked iris transillumination defects, peripheral anterior synechiae and corectopia and a grossly cupped disc.

9. A 2-year-old boy enters your cubicle and he is photophobic. He is being followed up frequently for persistent epithelial defects. Amongst the other signs, you notice that he has nystagmus and an epibulbar dermoid. On fundoscopy he has hypolastic maculae and optic discs. He is systemically well.

Theme: Landmark studies

Options
A   Early Manifest Glaucoma Study
B   Advanced Glaucoma Intervention Study
C   Ocular Hypertension Treatment Trial
D   5-FU Trial
E   Collaborative Initial Glaucoma Treatment Study
F   None of the above

For each of the scenarios below, select the single most relevant trial from the list above. Each option may be used once, more than once or not at all.

10.   This multicentred randomized controlled trial recruited patients with signs of glaucoma previously untreated. (Patients with advanced glaucomatous changes were excluded.) They were randomized to a treatment arm and no treatment arm. Treatment delayed progression of glaucoma.

11.   Newly diagnosed open angle glaucoma patients were randomized into one of two treatment arms: (i) medical treatment followed by laser trabeculoplasty followed by trabeculectomy; (ii) trabeculectomy as first-line treatment. Interim results did not show that trabeculectomy as first-line treatment should supersede medical treatment.

12.   A 40-year-old Afro-Carribean man has had an intraocular pressure of 25 mmHg, he has a thin central cornea, vC:D ratio of 0.5 in both eyes and on Humphrey field analysis in the right eye nasal field loss. Which of the above trials suggest that such a patient requires topical treatment.

Theme: Surgical/laser treatment

Options
A   180 degrees ciliary body cyclodiode
B   Argon laser trabeculoplasty
C   Trabeculectomy with 5-FU
D   Trabeculectomy with mitomycin C
E   Glaucoma drainage tube
F   Trabeculectomy, phakoemulsification and intraocular lens insertion

For each of the clinical scenarios below, select the single most likely procedure from the list above. Each option may be used once, more than once or not at all.

13.   A 35-year-old man has a history of chronic uveitis. In his left eye he has progressive visual field changes, intraocular pressure of 26 mmHg, vC:D of 0.7. He has an early posterior subcapsular cataract. He is on maximal medical treatment including oral acetazolamide. Which of the above procedures would be most appropriate for him?

14.   A 75-year-old man had a central retinal vein occlusion 1 year ago. He recently developed neovascular glaucoma and requires oral diamox. His vision is PL in that eye. Which of the above procedures would be most appropriate for him?

15.   A 60-year-old Afro-Caribbean woman has longstanding primary open angle glaucoma in both eyes. She is on four different drops to lower her intraocular pressure. In her right eye she has noticed that her vision is subjectively worse over the past 6 months. Visual fields show progression in her right eye. Which of the above procedures would be most appropriate for her?

Theme: What is the glaucoma diagnosis?

Options
A   Ocular hypertension
B   Primary open angle glaucoma
C   Normal tension glaucoma
D   Narrow angle glaucoma
E   Plateau iris
F   Angle recession glaucoma

For each of the clinical scenarios below, select the single most likely diagnosis from the list above. Each option may be used once, more than once or not at all.

16.   A 65-year-old Caucasian woman complains of blurred vision in her right eye. She has no past ocular history. She has a family history of glaucoma. On examination there is no corneal opacity, no cataract, no abnormality of vitreous, no macular abnormality, retinal vasculature and retina is healthy. Her intraocular pressure is OD 28 mmHg and OS 18 mmHg. The right optic disc has superior rim thinning and she has a marked right inferior arcuate defect that encroaches fixation. Gonioscopy shows normal angle structures in both eyes and Schaffer grade 4.

17.   A 55-year-old man is referred by his optician for raised intraocular pressures in both eyes. He has no past medical or family history. His intraocular pressures are OD 27 mmHg and OS 25 mmHg. Gonioscopy reveals normal angle structures and Schaffer grading of 3. Pachymetry in the right eye is 499 μm and left eye 510 μm. He has a vC : D ratio of 0.6 in both eyes. There is no focal rim abnormlity. He has normal visual fields.

18.   A 40-year-old man attends clinic complaining of unilateral gradual visual loss noticeable over the period of a year. His intraocular pressure is 30 mmHg. He has marked glaucomatous field loss in the same eye. On gonioscopy there is a 180 degrees area of uneven iris insertion and torn iris processes. This area also reveals an area of widened ciliary band. The other eye has normal angle structures. His optic disc in the affected eye has a cup:disc ratio of 0.8 and the other eye 0.4. On further questioning he recalls a blunt trauma to that eye 20 years ago.

Theme: What is the mechanism of raised intraocular pressure?

Options
A   Anterior rotation of ciliary body
B   Pigment occluding trabeculum and toxicity of trabecular meshwork
C   Raised episcleral venous pressure
D   Iris occluding trabecular meshwork
E   Contraction of fibrovascular membrane over angle structures
F   Anterior displacement of vitreous, ciliary processes and intraocular lens.

For each of the clinical scenarios below, select the single most likely pathology that has occurred from the list above. Each option may be used once, more than once or not at all.

19.   A 25-year-old man complains of intermittent blurring of vision particularly after exercise. On examination he has Krukenberg's spindle, mid peripheral iris transillumination defects, Sampolesi's line on gonioscopy and pigment deposition on peripheral anterior capsule of crystalline lens. His intraocular pressure is 28 mmHg in the right eye and 30 mmHg in the left eye. The optic discs in both eyes are healthy and there is no visual field defect.

20.   A 45-year-old man complains of intermittent pain and haloes. He is phakic in both eyes and has intraocular pressures of 30 mmHg in both eyes. Van Herrick assessment of the anterior chamber is grade 3. Gonioscopy shows angle crowding, iris is inserted anteriorly and indentation gonioscopy does not open the angle. Visual fields are normal.

21.   A 45-year-old woman with a history of rheumatoid arthritis attends casualty with a 1-day history of an extremely sore and red left eye. She has a history of anterior scleritis in her right eye. On examination her vision has reduced to 6/36 in the left eye. There is microcystic oedema of the cornea, her intraocular pressure is 55 mmHg OS. The anterior chamber is shallow. She is phakic. A B-scan shows thickening of the posterior sclera.

Theme: Investigating glaucoma

Options
A   HRT (Heidelberg retinal tomograph)
B   GDx nerve fibre layer analyser
C   OCT (optical coherence tomography)
D   Pachymetry
E   SITA visual field (Swedish international threshold algorithmn)
F   Optic disc photograph

For each of the clinical scenarios below, select the single most useful investigative instrument from the list above. Each option may be used once, more than once or not at all.

22.   This imaging system gives high resolution cross-sectional images of the retina. It can potentially be used in glaucoma for retinal nerve fibre layer thickness analysis. The image acquired is an intensity map of light back scattered or reflected from tissue structures compared to light reflected from the reference mirror.

23.   This instrument is a confocal laser scanning system that is able to give 3D images of different layers of the disc and retina. Its main uses are in optic nerve head analysis in glaucoma and retinal thickness in macular oedema. It is able to give quantitative results.

24.   As a result of the Ocular Hypertension Treatment Trial many eye units have acquired this instrument to work up a subgroup of patients to assess their risk of developing glaucoma.

Theme: Complications of a trabeculectomy

Options
A   Suprachoroidal haemorrhage
B   Encysted bleb ('ring of steel')
C   Blebitis
D   'Wipe-out'
E   Malignant glaucoma
F   Leaking bleb

For each of the clinical scenarios below, select the single most likely complication from the list above. Each option may be used once, more than once or not at all.

25.   A patient presents to casualty with a sticky and red eye. He has had two trabeculectomies in that eye and the second with mitomycin C. On examination the conjunctiva and bleb are injected. The bleb has a milky white appearance. The anterior chamber is deep, there are 2+ cells and flare. The vitreous is quiet. The intraocular pressure is 14 mmHg. Conjunctival swabs are taken and he is admitted for intensive medical treatment and frequent monitoring.

26.   A patient with a trabeculectomy is followed up in clinic and it is discovered that her intraocular pressure is increasing. On careful slit-lamp examination of the bleb you see a dome of episcleral scar tissue. This requires needling to create a fistula.

27.   A patient is followed up in glaucoma clinic 1 week postop. and has an intraocular pressure of 5 mmHg. The anterior chamber is deep. There are choroidal folds and maculopathy on fundoscopy.

Theme: Medical therapy

Options
A   Latanoprost
B   Pilocarpine
C   Timolol
D   Brimonidine
E   Glycerol
F   Acetazolamide

For each of the clinical scenarios below, select the single most suitable drug for treatment from the list above. Each option may be used once, more than once or not at all.

28.   A 56-year-old patient presents to casualty with an intraocular pressure of 56 mmHg in her left eye. The cornea is very cloudy, the anterior chamber is flat, there is iris bombe and she is phakic with nuclear sclerosis. Gonioscopy shows a closed angle. She was given intravenous diamox 500 mg 2 hours ago. This has not lowered the intraocular pressure. Which of the above would you try next?

29.   You follow up a patient in clinic. On the last visit their medical treatment was increased from two drops to three. Since the last visit he was admitted under the cardiologists to investigate his shortness of breath. They did not find a cause and he forgot to mention that he was taking glaucoma drops. Which of the above caused his shortness of breath?

30.   A 35-year-old who is a low hyperope attends clinic. His anterior chamber depth is normal. His intraocular pressure is 16 mmHg in both eyes. On gonioscopy there is angle crowding, iris is inserted anteriorly and is in contact with the trabecular meshwork and angles don't open on indentation goniscopy. Laser peripheral iridotomies will not change the iris configuration. Which of the above should be used?

Chapter 5

Uveitis – EMQs

- This chapter consists of 30 extended matching questions.
- Questions consist of a theme, a list of options, an instruction and a variable number of clinical situations.
- For each of the clinical situations, you should choose the **single most likely option** according to the instruction.
- It is possible for one option to be the answer to more than one of the clinical situations.

Chapter 5: Uveitis EMQs

Theme: HLA associations

Options
A A29
B B5
C B7
D Bw44
E B27
F DR3

For each of the clinical scenarios below, select the single most likely HLA association from the list above. Each option may be used once, more than once or not at all.

1. A young Caucasian patient presents with bilateral gradual reduction in vision. Her vision in the right eye is 6/18 and in the left eye 6/24. On examination the positive findings are a mild anterior chamber activity, vitritis, subfoveal choroidal neovascular membrane and multifocal choroiditis.

2. You are following up a 9-year-old child in clinic who had a previous drug reaction to a sulfonamide that has left her with marked lid and ocular surface abnormalities. She has upper and lower lid trichiasis for which she has had previous anterior lamellar repositioning. She has marked ankyloblepharon and inferior fornix shortening due to symblepharon. There is 360 degrees of peripheral corneal vascularization and bilateral pannus. She has secondary dry eyes and suffers frequent episodes of microbial keratitis. She uses topical antibiotics and retinoic acid.

3. A 48-year-old woman attends casualty with bilateral blurry vision that has come on over a period of a week or so. Her visual acuity is OD 6/36 ua OS 6/24 ua. She has mild anterior chamber activity, moderate vitritis, optic disc swelling, cystoid macular oedema, midperipheral chorioretinal lesions, retinal vasculitis and an area of subretinal neovascular membrane in the right eye. There are no systemic features.

Theme: Intermediate uveitis

Options
A   Multiple sclerosis
B   Sarcoidosis
C   Syphilis
D   Lyme disease
E   Lymphoma
F   Idiopathic

For each of the clinical scenarios below, select the single most likely diagnosis from the list above. Each option may be used once, more than once or not at all.

4. A middle-aged man has returned from a holiday in mid-west United States a few weeks ago. He complains of recovering from a flu-like illness on his return and presents to eye casualty with bilateral blurred vision and excruciating headaches. On examination he has a scar on his arm that looks like an insect bite in the middle surrounded by a bright circular red ring. He has bilateral conjunctivitis, papillitis and choroiditis. After discussion with your consultant you send off serology. After discussion with physicians he is treated with oral doxycycline and referred to neurologists. You arrange to see him next week.

5. An Afro-Caribbean woman in her 50s presents to uveitis clinic with bilateral blurred vision and a history of seizures and chronic shortness of breath. She has an inflamed anterior chamber, the vitreous has 2+ cells, there are snowballs and inferior snowbanking associated with vitreous traction. In the posterior pole she has chronic changes associated with macular oedema (this is confirmed on OCT). You decide to discuss the management of her macular oedema with your consultant.

6. A young woman with a history of previous sudden visual loss with complete recovery and recent pins-and-needles in both her feet attends for routine follow-up in the uveitis clinic. On examination she has visual acuity of 6/6 and 6/5. There is minimal anterior segment inflammation. She has slight posterior capsular opacification. There are cells +1 in the anterior vitreous, the right disc has mild pallor, there is no macular oedema, however there is bilateral peripheral venous sheathing. She is advised to continue topical steroid treatment and she will be reviewed again in a couple of weeks.

Theme: Uveitis

Options
A   HLA A29
B   Intermediate uveitis
C   Anterior uveitis
D   Panuveitis
E   HLA B51
F   Multifocal choroiditis

For each of the clinical scenarios below, select the single most likely diagnosis from the list above. Each option may be used once, more than once or not at all.

7. A young Turkish man presents with unilateral red eye and blurred vision. His vision is 6/36. In his anterior chamber he has a hypopyon, there is moderate vitritis, cystoid macular oedema, branch retinal vein occlusion and extensive peripheral vasculitis involving both arteries and veins.

8. A 7-year-old boy presents with joint pains in both knees. He complains of a 1-year history of intermittent sore eyes and his vision is 6/36 in his right eye and 6/9 in his left eye. He has 3+ cells in both anterior chambers and 1+ cells in both anterior vitreous. In his right eye he has cystoid macular oedema.

9. A 45-year-old woman complains of bilateral blurring of vision and floaters. On examination she has minimal anterior segment inflammation, moderate vitritis, there is blurring of the disc margins due to multiple scattered chorioretinal creamy white lesions that radiate away from the disc towards the equator. There is macular oedema and peripheral vasculitis

Theme: Inflammatory conditions of the choroid and retina

Options
A   Serpiginous choroidopathy
B   Punctate inner choroidopathy
C   Acute posterior multifocal placoid pigment epitheliopathy
D   Vogt–Koyanagi–Harada disease
E   Multiple evanescent white dot syndrome
F   Acute retinal pigment epitheliitis (Krill's disease)

For each of the clinical scenarios below, select the single most likely diagnosis from the list above. Each option may be used once, more than once or not at all.

10.   As you walk into the medical retina clinic you walk past a young woman, sitting in the waiting area, who is wearing concave glasses. You 'second-guess' her diagnosis before calling her in. As you read the notes your suspicion is confirmed, She is attending because a recent flare up resulted in a subretinal neovascular membrane associated with a lesion. There are multiple well-defined punched out depigmented lesions (between 100 and 300 µm) mainly within the vascular arcades in both posterior poles.

11.   A young man in his mid-20s is seen in uveitis clinic. He has bilateral blurred vision and complains of distortion. On examination the anterior chamber is quiet and there is a mild vitritis. He has lesions in both posterior poles. There are multiple creamy white lesions (500–2500 µm) and there are older lesions with varying degrees of pigmentary mottling. Fluorescein angiography is characteristic, it shows absent early choroidal fluorescence followed by late staining. Indocyanine green angiography shows abnormal delayed choroidal flow under the placoid lesions.

12.   A healthy young woman aged 25 years has a history of unilateral acute onset blurring of vision. On examination there is enlargement of the blind spot and a vision of 6/60. There are multiple discrete small white lesions (100–200 µm) at the level of the retinal pigment epithelium. On fluorescein angiography these lesions hyperfluoresce early and stain late. She has a good prognosis, doesn't require treatment and is advised that this is unlikely to recur, but is warned that some patients have a tendency to progress to photopsia associated with unusual visual field loss patterns (AZOOR).

Theme: Posterior uveitis

Options
A   Toxoplasma chorioretinitis
B   Vogt–Koyanagi–Harada syndrome
C   Behçet's
D   Sympathetic ophthalmitis
E   Sarcoidosis
F   Associated with systemic lupus erythematosus

For each of the clinical scenarios below, select the single most likely diagnosis from the list above. Each option may be used once, more than once or not at all.

13.   A 25-year-old Japanese man presents with tinnitus, headaches and reduction in his vision. On examination he has mid anterior segment inflammation in his right eye. He has mild vitritis, a swollen and hypcracmic disc, serous retinal elevation in the posterior pole and periphery, a wide area of multiple spotty, deep chorioretinal creamy-white lesions. There is no other cranial nerve abnormality or focal neurology. There is no skin abnormality. He is treated with high dose steroid and topical steroids in the first instance.

14.   You review a 35-year-old woman in clinic. She has a systemic history of malar rash, arthritis and renal problems. Examining her posterior segment she has marked arteriolar narrowing, multiple areas of both branch retinal and vein occlusion with peripheral closure on fluorescein angiography. There are multiple cotton wool spots and hard exudates. She also has a history of anterior scleritis. She has been on long-term immunosuppression.

15.   A 28-year-old Japanese woman has a history of aphthous ulcers and erythema nodosum. Examining her posterior segment she has an area of branch retinal artery and vein occlusion with retinal oedema and haemorrhage – this is an occlusive vasculitis. There are multiple areas of previous venous occlusion. There is also overlying vitreous haze due to vitritis. She is currently on both oral prednisolone and azathioprine.

Theme: Treatment options in uveitis

Options
A   Argon laser photocoagulation
B   Posterior subtenons triamcinolone
C   Intravitreal steroid
D   Intravenous gangciclovir
E   Anterior chamber TPA (tissue plasminogen activator)
F   Vitrectomy

For each of the clinical scenarios below, select the single most likely therapy from the list above. Each option may be used once, more than once or not at all.

16.   A 32-year-old woman from Somalia who has been living in the UK for 7 months attends for follow-up in the uveitis clinic because she has confluent areas of full thickness necrotizing retinitis with haemorrhage and associated vasculitis and an overlying minimal vitritis. She has CD4+ count of less than 50 cells/µl.

17.   A 29-year-old man from India who has been living in the UK for 8 months attends the uveitis clinic with unilateral blurring of vision. On examination he has very little anterior chamber activity. He has marked disc new vessels retinal and vitreous haemorrhage. In the periphery there is retinal vascular sheathing (periphlebitis) and ghost vessels and an equatorial area of new vessels. Flourescein angiography shows peripheral ischaemia.

18.   A young woman with known multiple sclerosis attends the uveitis clinic for a longstanding history of floaters and recent blurring of vision in her right eye. On examination she has 1+ cells and flare in the right anterior chamber, there are cells in the anterior vitreous and inferior snowballs, there is no snowbanking. She has cystoid macular oedema confirmed on OCT.

Theme: Surgical interventions in uveitic eyes

Options
A   Chelation with EDTA
B   Subfoveal membranectomy
C   Seton drainage
D   Lensectomy with pars plana vitrectomy
E   Phakoemulsification and PMMA lens implant
F   Phakoemulsification and acrylic lens implant

For each of the clinical scenarios below, select the single most likely surgical intervention from the list above. Each option may be used once, more than once or not at all.

19.   An 18-year-old girl has a history of recurrent bilateral anterior uveitis and arthritis in her knees and elbows. She is ANA+ve, rheumatoid factor –ve and HLA B27–ve. Her chronic uveitis has resulted in bilateral posterior subcapsular cataracts and raised intraocular pressure not controllable on maximal medical therapy. What is her next option?

20.   A man from Missisippi, USA complains of right blurred vision that has progressed over the past few weeks. On examination the anterior chamber is quiet, there is minimal vitritis. At the posterior pole there are multiple punched out chorioretinal lesions and at the macula there is one associated with a subretinal neovascular membrane confirmed on fluorescein angiography. It is decided not to treat this with focal argon laser.

21.   A woman with ocular and pulmonary sarcoidosis attends for follow-up. She has completed a tapering regime of g Maxidex in her left eye. On examination there is peripheral band keratopathy, old keratic precipitates, anterior chamber flare, a posterior subcapsular cataract, no vitritis and no cystoid macular oedema. What are her options to improve her vision?

Theme: Anterior uveitis

Options
A   Juvenile idiopathic arthritis
B   HLA B27 associated anterior uveitis
C   Reiter's syndrome
D   Fuch's heterochromic cyclitis
E   Posner–Schlossman syndrome
F   Psoriatic arthritis

For each of the clinical scenarios below, select the single most likely diagnosis from the list above. Each option may be used once, more than once or not at all.

22.   A 30-year-old man who is diagnosed with unilateral anterior uveitis has had 20 episodes since the age of 25. He is HLA B27+ve. He is otherwise fit and well. He has had an episode of macular oedema recently that responded well to posterior subtenons triamcinolone visually but his intraocular pressure is 40 mmHg and requires anti-hypertensive ocular treatment.

23.   A 55-year-old woman presents to casualty with a 1-month history of an ache in her left eye with mild redness and a 5-day history of headache. On examination she has 1+ cells and flare in her anterior chamber. Her intraocular pressure is 52 mmHg in left eye and 18 mmHg in right eye. Gonioscopy shows wide open angles, there are no peripheral anterior synechiae. Looking through her casualty card this has happened before about 6 months ago and she responded to systemic, topical antihypertensives and topical steroids.

24.   A young man presents to casualty with a unilateral red and watery eye. On examination he has conjunctivitis, non-granulomatous anterior uveitis. He has suffered recently from urethral discharge. There are no abnormalities of his hands or feet. He is treated with topical steroids and referred to a physician.

Theme: Systemic therapy in inflammatory conditions

Options
A   Cyclosporin
B   Cyclophosphamide
C   Clindamycin
D   High dose intravenous steroid
E   Azathioprine
F   Dapsone

For each of the clinical scenarios below, select the single most suitable systemic therapy from the list above. Each option may be used once, more than once or not at all.

25.   A 35-year-old man presents with an exquisitely painful and red left eye and blocked nose. On examination he has marked congestion of episcleral vessels, there is no associated nodule. He has a past medical history of chronic renal problems but cannot remember what the renal diagnosis is.

26.   An elderly Caucasian lady presents with bilateral sore eyes. On examination she has bilateral mild conjunctival injection, trichiasis, symblepharon, forniceal shortening, increased tear break-up time. Everting the lids reveals marked subepithelial fibrosis. There is no surface keratinization. The anterior chamber is quiet.

27.   A pregnant Brazilian woman presents to casualty with a 2-day history of blurry vision in her right eye and an increase in floaters. On examination she has 2+ cells in her anterior chamber and marked vitritis with a fluffy yellow-white lesion at the posterior pole just inferior to the superior arcade a disc diameter from the optic disc. This lesion is adjacent to a large chorioretinal scar with a pigmentary edge.

Theme: Uveitis and systemic disease

Options
A Still's disease
B Pauciarticular juvenile rheumatoid arthritis
C Systemic lupus erythematosus
D Wegener's granulomatosis
E Rheumatoid arthritis
F Ankylosing spondylitis

For each of the clinical scenarios below, select the single most likely diagnosis from the list above. Each option may be used once, more than once or not at all.

28. A young girl of 8 suffers from joint pain in both knees and both elbows. She is ANA+ve, rheumatoid factor negative and HLA B27–ve. She has had frequent recurrent anterior uveitis.

29. A young man is seronegative, ANA–ve and HLA B27+ve. He suffers from spinal pain worse at rest and at night than with activity. He also suffers from pain radiating down the back of his thigh and buttock. In addition he suffers from aortic regurgitation.

30. A man of 31 years suffers with chronic cough and haemoptysis and dyspnoea. He has regular renal dialyses as he has a history of necrotizing glomerulonephritis. His c-ANCA levels are currently low. He presents to the eye clinic with unilateral reduction in vision and proptosis.

Chapter 6

Medical Retina – EMQs

- This chapter consists of 60 extended matching questions.
- Questions consist of a theme, a list of options, an instruction and a variable number of clinical situations.
- For each of the clinical situations, you should choose the **single most likely option** according to the instruction.
- It is possible for one option to be the answer to more than one of the clinical situations.

Theme: Clinical trials in the management of diabetic retinopathy

Options
A   Diabetic Retinopathy Study
B   Early Treatment of Diabetic Retinopathy Study
C   Diabetic Retinopathy Vitrectomy Study
D   Diabetic Controls and Complications Trial
E   UKPDS
F   None of the above

For each of the clinical trials below, select the single most likely trial from the list above. Each option may be used once, more than once or not at all.

1. Which trial assessed the effect of panretinal photocoagulation on proliferative diabetic retinopathy? Patients recruited had proliferative or severe non-proliferative diabetic retinopathy in both eyes. One eye was treated and compared to the fellow non-treated eye. At 5 years there was a 50% reduction in severe visual loss in treated eyes compared to non-treated eyes. Treated eyes with high-risk proliferative diabetic retinopathy achieved the greatest benefit. As a result early panretinal photocoagulation is recommended for high-risk proliferative diabetic retinopathy.

2. This trial showed type 1 diabetics with vitreous haemorrhage or advanced proliferative diabetic retinopathy benefited from early vitrectomy.

3. This trial showed that intensive control of blood glucose versus normal control delays onset and slows progression of diabetic retinopathy, reduces the risk of developing neuropathy and albuminuria.

Theme: ETDRS classification of diabetic retinopathy

Options
A   Mild non-proliferative diabetic retinopathy
B   Moderate non-proliferative diabetic retinopathy
C   Severe non-proliferative diabetic retinopathy
D   Early proliferative diabetic retinopathy
E   High-risk proliferative diabetic retinopathy
F   Advanced proliferative diabetic retinopathy

For each of the clinical scenarios below, select the single most likely diagnostic classification from the list above. Each option may be used once, more than once or not at all.

4.   A 45-year-old Indian man with type 1 diabetes has greater than a disc area of NVD, and two quadrants of NVE. There is intragel and subretinal vitreous haemorrhage. There is also an area of traction just inferior to the macula. He has had panretinal photocoagulation in both eyes.

5.   A 50-year-old Caucasian woman is a type 2 diabetic. She has four quadrants of blot haemorrhages, two quadrants of venous beading and one quadrant of intraretinal microvascular aneurysms in both eyes.

6.   A 20-year-old woman is a type 1 diabetic. She has an area of NVE less than one-quarter disc area just beneath the inferior vascular arcade and a small frond of flat new vessels less than one-quarter of a disc diameter.

Theme: Managing diabetic retinopathy I

Options
A   Grid laser
B   Focal laser
C   Vitrectomy
D   Panretinal photocoagulation
E   Observe 3-monthly intervals
F   Intravitreal triamcinolone

For each of the clinical scenarios below, select the single most suitable treatment from the list above. Each option may be used once, more than once or not at all.

7. A 48-year-old man has bilateral treated proliferative diabetic retinopathy. His vision in his right eye is 6/18 and in his left eye 6/9 corrected. Clinically there is retinal thickening greater than one disc area in size and one disc diameter from the fovea. What would you do next?

8. A 53-year-old man is type 2 diabetic with poor glycaemic control. He has bilateral NVD greater than one-half disc area, bilateral peripheral new vessels in two quadrants and in the right eye inferior preretinal haemorrhage. There are also hard exudates with associated retinal thickening within 500 μm of the fovea. What would you do next?

9. A 21-year-old type 1 diabetic has treated proliferative diabetic retinopathy. Her vision has become blurred since her last visit 6 months ago. She has hard exudates less than 500 μm from fovea and associated retinal thickening. There are two other areas of retinal oedema within 500 μm from fovea with associated microaneurysms.

Theme: Managing diabetic retinopathy II

Options
A   Fill-in panretinal photocoagulation
B   Delamination and vitrectomy
C   Intravitreal triamcinolone
D   Sector panretinal photocoagulation
E   Argon grid laser
F   None of the above

For each of the clinical scenarios below, select the single most suitable treatment from the list above. Each option may be used once, more than once or not at all.

10.   A type 1 diabetic woman on fundoscopy has fresh NVD (non-clubbed vessel ends) protruding from the disc into the vitreous cavity. There is no vitreous haemorrhage. She has previously had 360 degree panretinal photocoagulation.

11.   A diabetic man on fundoscopy has dot and blot haemorrhages in three quadrants. At the right macula he has had macular oedema for over 1 year and has had three grid treatments. His vision in the right eye is 6/24.

12.   A 55-year-old woman has had bilateral treated proliferative diabetic retinopathy with several fill-in panretinal photocoagulations too. In the right eye there is a vitreous haemorrhage that has not cleared after 8 months and now she has had a re-bleed.

Theme: Vein occlusion

Options
A   Central retinal vein occlusion study
B   Branch retinal vein occlusion study
C   Panretinal photocoagulation
D   Sector panretinal photocoagulation
E   Focal/grid laser
F   None of the above

For each of the clinical scenarios below, select the single most likely study from the list above. Each option may be used once, more than once or not at all.

13.   This study showed that panretinal photocoagulation prior to the onset of new vessels elsewhere or new vessels at the disc is necessary as a prophylactic measure to prevent rubeosis.

14.   Five months ago a 60-year-old man experienced a sudden decrease in vision in his left eye down to 6/60. Now he has new vessels at the disc and 360 degrees of new vessels at the pupillary margin and also in two quadrants on gonioscopy. The retinal haemorrhage at the posterior pole has nearly resolved. There is marked vascular tortuosity and chronic macular oedema. Fluorescein angiography reveals marked capillary dropout at the macula.

15.   A 58-year-old man has a 3-month history of superotemporal branch retinal vein occlusion. He has macular oedema and 6/18 vision in the same eye. There are associated new vessels and capillary non-perfusion on fluorescein angiography in the area of branch vein occlusion.

Theme: Vascular retinopathy

Options
A   Sickle cell proliferative retinopathy
B   Sickle cell non-proliferative retinopathy
C   Eale's disease
D   Coat's disease
E   Acute hypertensive retinopathy
F   None of the above

For each of the clinical scenarios below, select the single most likely diagnosis from the list above. Each option may be used once, more than once or not at all.

16.   A 31-year-old Afro-Caribbean man has a history of acute admissions for blood transfusions and intravenous fluids. On fundal examination there is a cup : disc ratio of 0.5 with a healthy rim. There is no abnormality at the macula. In the periphery there is venous tortuosity, arteriolar narrowing and peripheral chorioretinal scars (black sunbursts). There is an area of ghost vessels due to a previous arteriolar occlusion.

17.   A 21-year-old Indian man has a 7-month history of reduced vision in his right eye. The left is amblyopic. On examination he has new vessels at the disc and peripheral ischaemia due to a branch retinal vein occlusion and branch retinal arterial occlusion. There are peripheral new vessels (sea-fan configuration) and areas of preretinal haemorrhage with red blood cells in the vitreous.

18.   A 60-year-old man with no significant past medical history presents with a 1-week history of headaches and a blurred disc, tortuous vessels and marked haemorrhagic fundus in the right eye. The left eye has a normal disc with no spontaneous venous pulsation. There is marked arteriovenous nipping of first order vessels.

Theme: Age-related macular degeneration

Options
A Focal argon laser
B Photodynamic therapy
C Ocuvite
D Low vision aids
E None of the above

For each of the clinical scenarios below, select the single most suitable therapy from the list above. Each option may be used once, more than once or not at all.

19. A 60-year-old man has disciform scars and drusen in both the posterior poles. His visual acuity is 1/60 in his right eye and hand movements in the left eye.

20. A 70-year-old male smoker has a disciform scar in one eye and a soft confluent drusen in the other eye. His vision is 2/60 in the right eye and 6/9 in the left eye.

21. A 60-year-old with bilateral macular drusen has visual acuity of 6/36 in his right eye and on fluorescein a classic membrane with no occult component.

Theme: Vitreous haemorrhage

Options
A   Terson's syndrome
B   Age-related macular degeneration
C   Posterior vitreous detachment
D   Eale's disease
E   Familial exudative vitreo-retinopathy
F   Retinal telangiectasia

For each of the clinical scenarios below, select the single most likely diagnosis from the list above. Each option may be used once, more than once or not at all.

22.   A 1-year-old boy has bilateral poor vision in both eyes and a sensory esotropia. He is systemically well. On examination of the anterior segment he has bilateral posterior subcapsular cataracts. The posterior pole has macular thickening with serous fluid, hard exudates. The retinal capillaries are distorted with dragging of the macula and there is fibrovascular proliferation temporally.

23.   A 60-year-old Caucasian woman has bilateral soft drusen. Inspecting the vitreous in downgaze there are red blood cells. On inspection in the same eye there is an area of thickening adjacent to the fovea.

24.   Following a road traffic accident a 40-year-old man who was knocked off his motorbike suffered a subdural haemorrhage. He complains of bilateral reduction in vision following flashing lights. On examination he has scattered preretinal haemorrhages in the peripapillary region. There are also scattered subretinal haemorrhages and a dense vitreous haemorrhage.

Theme: Investigations

Options

A   Ocular coherence tomography
B   Doppler carotid ultrasound
C   Haemoglobin electrophoresis
D   Indo-cyanine-green angiogram
E   Antiphospholipid antibodies (anticardiolipin antibody and lupus anti-coagulant)
F   None of the above

For each of the clinical scenarios below, select the single most suitable investigative tool from the list above. Each option may be used once, more than once or not at all.

25.   A 25-year-old woman with a history of two previous miscarriages presents to casualty with a unilateral sudden painless loss of vision. On examination anterior segment is unremarkable and in the fundus there is marked vascular tortuosity, scattered preretinal haemorrhages and mild disc swelling. Blood pressure is normal. Which of the above would explain her history?

26.   A 65-year-old man presents with a unilateral red eye, corneal oedema, anterior chamber flare, intraocular pressure is normal. In the fundus there is marked vascular tortuosity, venous dilatation, retinal haemorrhages, microaneurysms and a swollen disc. ESR is normal. Which of the above will give essential information, as his condition will have serious implications regarding his 5-year mortality rate?

27.   An Afro-Caribbean woman presents with a hemi-arterial occlusion. There is no evidence of retinal arterial emboli. There is, however, peripheral venous attenuation, sea-fan shaped vessels and a pigmentary patch called a 'sun-burst'. She is referred to physicians for urgent blood transfusion. Which of the above will aid systemic diagnosis?

Theme: Fluorescein angiogram I

Options
A   Central serous retinopathy
B   Ocular ischaemic syndrome
C   Subretinal neovascular membrane with occult
D   Subretinal neovascular membrane with no occult
E   Macular oedema secondary to diabetes mellitus
F   Irvine–Gass syndrome

For each of the clinical scenarios below, select the single most likely diagnosis from the list above. Each option may be used once, more than once or not at all.

28.   A 25-year-old asthmatic male banker complains of blurred, dimmed vision, metamorphopsia. His vision is 6/18 and this improves with a +1 D lens. On fundal examination there is a dome-shaped elevation at the macula with no associated haemorrhage or hard exudates.

29.   One week post phako a diabetic patient is reviewed. He complains his vision is worse before than preoperatively. He has retinal thickening at the macula and a dull foveal reflex.

30.   A 70-year-old patient describes a sudden reduction in unilateral vision. Fluorescein angiogram shows delayed choroidal filling and a delayed arteriole to venous transit time. Late phase shows arteriolar staining.

Theme: Fluorescein angiogram II

Options
A   Stargardt's disease
B   Best's disease
C   Adult vitelliform cyst
D   Presumed ocular histoplasmosis
E   Acute Vogt–Koyanagi–Harada syndrome
F   Retinal pigment epithelial detachment

For each of the clinical scenarios below, select the single most likely diagnosis from the list above. Each option may be used once, more than once or not at all.

31.   During the early phase there is a dark fundus due to blockage of background choroidal fluorescence. There are numerous hyperfluorescent lesions within the macular area.

32.   During the early phase the choroid looks dark. There is a wider than normal hypofluorescent area at the fovea. Then in the venous phase a few spots begin to appear at the fovea and macula and then increase in number. In the late phase there is staining that resembles a scrambled egg.

33.   In the choroidal to early arterial phase there are multiple punctate hypofluorescent dots followed by patchy areas of irregular hyperfluorescence. In the late phase the dye pools into well-defined areas of the inner retina.

Theme: Hereditary retina I

Options

A   Gyrate atrophy
B   Retinitis pigmentosa
C   Congenital stationary night blindness
D   Stargardt's macular dystrophy
E   North Carolina dystrophy
F   None of the above

For each of the clinical scenarios below, select the single most likely diagnosis from the list above. Each option may be used once, more than once or not at all.

34.   This condition is associated with a large increase in plasma, urine and CSF ornithine levels. It is an autosomal recessive condition that causes a deficiency in the enzyme ornithine keto-acid aminotransferase. Presentation occurs in early childhood with an increase in myopia, reduced peripheral fields and nyctalopia. Fundoscopy shows circular patches of chorioretinal atrophy in the mid and far periphery. These lesions become larger and coalesce. The retinal vessels are extremely attenuated and cystoid macular oedema develops. There is a flat EOG and ERG. Vitamin B_6 supplements help slow down disease progression.

35.   A 45-year-old woman attends clinic referred by her optician who has found bilateral yellow spots in the retina. On examination her vision is 6/24 right eye and 6/18 left eye. She is worried she is becoming blind, as her reduction in vision has occurred over 18 months. She has scattered lesions from the posterior pole to the far periphery that vary from oval to linear in shape. She has scarring at both foveae. ERG confirms the maculopathy plus a cone dystrophy and that the condition is non-progressive.

36.   A 38-year-old man on examination has a visual acuity of 6/18 in both eyes, bilateral posterior subcapsular cataracts, arteriolar attenuation, waxy disc pallor and a few retinal boney-spicule pigmentary changes and peripheral telangiectasia. He is on diamox for cystoid macular oedema.

Theme: A negative ERG

Options
A   Central retinal artery occlusion
B   Congenital stationary night blindness
C   Juvenile X-linked retinoschisis
D   MAR (melanoma associated retinopathy)
E   Quinine retinopathy
F   Birdshot chorioretinopathy

For each of the clinical scenarios below, select the single most likely diagnosis from the list above. Each option may be used once, more than once or not at all.

37.   A young man has been registered blind since birth. He has a dominantly inherited condition. His fundus has a normal appearance. Electroretinogram is diagnostic: there is a negative ERG which locates this to an inner nuclear layer abnormality; there is no rod-specific ERG and a flat pattern ERG.

38.   A young Caucasian from Australia has pale freckly skin. She complains of shimmering photopsia and in the last 6 months progressive increase in nyctalopia. There is no abnormality of the fundus. She has a negative ERG, no rod-specific ERG and a flat pattern ERG. This is diagnostic and she is referred to a dermatologist.

39.   A 73-year-old woman was referred by her optician with bilateral constricted fields. On fundal examination she has disc pallor and constricted vessels. The macula looks normal. She describes an event when she was 19 years old. She ingested a substance in order to abort a pregnancy, following which she suffered sudden onset blackout of vision that recovered a day later. She has a negative ERG, reduced pattern ERG. The ON-OFF response has a characteristic sawtooth pattern pathognomic of this condition.

Theme: Hereditary retina II

Options
A   Bardet–Biedl syndrome
B   Familial dominant drusen
C   Best vitelliform macular dystrophy
D   Usher's syndrome
E   Choroideraemia
F   Leber's congenital amaurosis

For each of the clinical scenarios below, select the single most likely diagnosis from the list above. Each option may be used once, more than once or not at all.

40.   A 7-year-old boy has difficulty seeing at night. There are no systemic abnormalities and no abnormality of the anterior segment. On fundal examination there is diffuse retinal pigment epithelium and choroidal atrophy with prominence of the intermediate and large choridal vacsulature. There is no abnormality of the optic discs or vasculature.

41.   A child of 24 months was referred by paediatricians because they are concerned he cannot see. He is deaf, has epilepsy, renal and endocrine dysfunction. The child rubs his eyes a lot according to the mother and on examination you see he has enophthalmos. On further examination he has absent direct and indirect light reflexes. He has optic disc pallor and attenuation of retinal arterioles, bull's eye maculopathy and peripheral chorioretinal atrophy.

42.   A 10-year-old is blind and profoundly deaf. She has abnormal vestibular function and marked peripheral pigmentary retinopathy.

Theme: Subretinal neovascular membrane

Options
A   Choroidal naevus
B   Presumed ocular histoplasmosis
C   Punctate inner choroidopathy
D   Myopia
E   Angioid streaks
F   Toxoplasmosis

For each of the clinical scenarios below, select the single most significant diagnosis from the list above. Each option may be used once, more than once or not at all.

43.   A young man wears concave glasses. He has tilted discs with peri-papillary atrophy, prominent choroidal vasculature and periph-eral lattice degeneration, and in one eye retinopexy scars from a peripheral superior U-tear.

44.   A tall man in his mid-30s with a high-arched palate, large hand span, total arm length longer than body height, mitral valve regurgitation and inguinal hernias complains of blurred vision. In both eyes he has red/brown lines radiating from the discs. These lines have irregular contours and are wider than the retinal vessels and are deep to the retina (break in Bruch's membrane). The lines end abruptly, posterior to the equator. In the right eye one of these lines in the macular area is associated with retinal thickening and haemorrhage. In the retinal periphery there is stippled pigmentary retinal mottling.

45.   You are in a fluorescein meeting and the next slide shows a colour fundus photograph. There is marked peripapillary atrophy around each optic disc. There are multifocal atrophic choroidal lesions pos-terior to the equator in both eyes. Each spot is around or less than half a disc diameter in size. They are yellow and some have a pig-mented border. There is disciform scarring in one eye. The vitreous is normal and there are no cells.

Theme: Acquired diseases affecting the macula

Options
A   Central serous retinopathy
B   Age-related macular degeneration
C   Presumed ocular histoplasmosis
D   Gronblad–Strandberg syndrome
E   Macula hole
F   Epiretinal membrane

For each of the clinical scenarios below, select the single most likely diagnosis from the list above. Each option may be used once, more than once or not at all.

46.   On fundoscopy you see dark red/brown bands radiating from the optic disc. These represent breaks at Bruch's membrane. A stippled area of retina called peau d'orange is seen temporally. At the disc there are drusen and peripapillary atrophy. There are associated skin lesion, yellow papules in the neck and antecubital fossa. There is accelerated atherosclerosis resulting in premature coronary artery disease. There is also associated gastrointestinal haemorrhage.

47.   A fundus fluorescein angiogram of a 35-year-old male banker shows an early hyperfluorescent spot that becomes larger and in the late venous phase the hyperfluorescent area ascends vertically forming a smoke stack appearance.

48.   A 40-year-old Caucasian woman presents with reduced vision and metamorphopsia in one eye due to an area of choroidal neovascularization at the macula. In both eyes she has punched out chorioretinal lesions in the mid periphery and juxtapapillary atrophic pigmentary changes. There is no vitreous inflammation.

Theme: Clinical trials

Options
A   AREDS – Age Related Eye Disease Study
B   CAPT – Complications of Age Related Macular Degeneration Prevention Trial
C   TAP – Treatment of Age Related Macular Degeneration with Photodynamic Therapy Study
D   VIP – Verteporforin Therapy Trial
E   MPS – Macular Photocoagulation Study
F   VIM – Visudyne in Minimally Classic Trial

For each of the clinical scenarios below, select the single most likely diagnosis from the list above. Each option may be used once, more than once or not at all.

49.   The objective of this study was to determine if photodynamic therapy with verteporforin can reduce the risk of visual loss in patients with subfoveal choroidal neovascularization (CNV) compared to sham treatment. The patients recruited had new or recurrent subfoveal CNV, a classic component, vision between 20/40 and 20/200, size <5400 µm and blood less than 50% of the lesion. At 1 and 2 years patients on the treated arm were less likely to suffer moderate visual loss compared to the placebo group. Subgroup analysis revealed the predominantly classic group rather than the minimally classic derived the most benefit.

50.   The objective of this study was to determine if photodynamic therapy with verteporforin can reduce the risk of visual loss in patients with subfoveal CNV compared to sham treatment. The patients enrolled had: (i) classic CNV +/– occult with visual acuities better than 20/40; (ii) occult membranes without a classic component; (iii) eyes with pathological myopia and subfoveal CNV. Outcomes at 2 years showed that the occult group did particularly well in the treated arm. The rates of moderate and severe visual loss were 49% and 21% in the treated arm compared to 75% and 48% in the placebo arm. An additional secondary outcome was that lesions larger than four disc areas in size should not be treated as they suffer a worse outcome with verteporforin treatment.

51. This study provides guidelines for the evaluation and management of patients with CNV secondary to age-related macular degeneration, ocular histoplasmosis and idiopathic choroidal neovascularization. Eyes with classic choroidal neovascularization had a better visual prognosis when treated with laser photocoagulation than the group under observation. These outcome data apply to all three conditions when the position of the neovascularization is extrafoveal or juxtafoveal, that is, when the CNV does not involve the centre of the fovea. Eyes receiving direct laser treatment to the fovea for new CNV **immediately** lost more visual acuity than eyes under observation alone. However, the amount of visual acuity loss in observed eyes increased to the level of loss in treated eyes **at 12 months** and exceeded the level thereafter. Eyes with smaller lesions and worse initial visual acuity had greater and earlier benefits from laser treatment. Eyes with large subfoveal neovascular lesions and good initial visual acuity are not good candidates for focal laser photocoagulation.

Theme: Systemic diseases associated with pigmentary retinopathy – autosomal dominant

Options
A   Alagille syndrome
B   Charcot–Marie–Tooth syndrome
C   Myotonic dystrophy
D   Waardenburg's syndrome
E   Olivopontocerebellar dysplasia syndrome
F   Oculodentodigital dysplasia syndrome

For each of the clinical scenarios below, select the single most likely diagnosis from the list above. Each option may be used once, more than once or not at all.

52.   Intrahepatic cholestatic syndrome, posterior embryotoxon, Axenfeld's anomaly, congenital heart disease, flattened facies and bridge of nose, myopia and pigmentary retinopathy.

53.   Hypertelorism, wide bridge of nose, cochlear deafness, white forelock, heterochromia iridis, poliosis, pigmentary disturbance of RPE.

54.   Retinal degeneration (peripheral/macular), cerebellar ataxia, possible external ophthalmoplegia.

Theme: Systemic disease associated with pigmentary retinopathy – autosomal recessive

Options
A   Bietti crystalline retinopathy
B   Friedreich's ataxia
C   Homocystinuria
D   Mannosidosis
E   Hurler's syndrome
F   Scheie's syndrome

For each of the clinical scenarios below, select the single most likely diagnosis from the list above. Each option may be used once, more than once or not at all.

55.   Coarse facies, aortic regurgitation, stiff joints, cloudy cornea, normal lifespan, normal intellect, pigmentary retinopathy.

56.   Spinocerebellar degeneration, limb incoordination, nerve deafness, retinal degeneration, optic atrophy.

57.   Yellow white crystals limited to the posterior pole at different retinal levels, round subretinal pigment deposition, confluent loss of choriocapillaris.

Theme: Miscellaneous

Options
A Parafoveal retinal telangiectasias
B Von Hippel–Lindau syndrome
C Eale's disease
D Ocular ischaemic syndrome
E Incontinentia pigmenti
F Retinopathy of prematurity

For each of the clinical scenarios below, select the single most likely diagnosis from the list above. Each option may be used once, more than once or not at all.

58. A 10-year-old boy has poor vision in both eyes with a right sensory exotropia. On fundoscopy he has a right dragged disc and macula. He was born at 26 weeks weighing 1200 g and required laser treatment in both eyes.

59. A 50-year-old woman describes loss of vision in one eye over a period of 6 weeks and she describes an aching pain around the ipsilateral orbital area. On examination she has iris neovascularization and anterior chamber flare. Intraocular pressure is normal. Fundoscopy shows narrowed retinal arterial, dilated retinal veins, retinal haemorrhages, microaneurysms and optic disc neovascularization. Fluorescein shows delayed choroidal filling, delayed arteriovenous transit time and late vascular staining. There is a past history of cerebrovascular accident.

60. This is a rare X-linked disorder that causes death in male fetuses. In females there is abnormal scaling, dryness of the skin, variable involvement of eye, teeth and central nervous system. Ocular involvement includes pigmentary abnormalities as well as peripheral retinal avascularity that leads to cicatricial retinal detachment.

Chapter 7

Vitreo-retinal Disorders – EMQs

- This chapter consists of 30 extended matching questions.
- Questions consist of a theme, a list of options, an instruction and a variable number of clinical situations.
- For each of the clinical situations, you should choose the **single most likely option** according to the instruction.
- It is possible for one option to be the answer to more than one of the clinical situations.

Theme: Vitrectomy for macular diseases

Options
A   Epiretinal membrane
B   Vitreo-macula traction syndrome
C   Idiopathic macula hole
D   Submacular haemorrhage
E   Subfoveal choroidal neovascularization
F   None of the above

For each of the clinical scenarios below, select the single most likely diagnosis from the list above. Each option may be used once, more than once or not at all.

1. On examination there is an incomplete posterior vitreous separation at the macula and optic nerve head. There is abnormal adherence of the vitreous to the posterior pole. The macula appears slightly tented anteriorly with a shallow detachment. The vision has dropped over 2 years from 6/12 to 6/36 due to cystoid macular oedema. The fluorescein angiogram shows disc leakage and diffuse accumulation of dye in the subsensory space, as a result of shallow detachment.

2. There is a full thickness defect at the macula greater than 400 μm. There is an associated posterior vitreous detachment. The visual acuity is 6/24. A fundus fluorescein angiogram would show a circular transmission defect as a result of the loss of xanthophyll, RPE depigmentation and atrophy. An OCT confirms the clinical findings.

3. A 60-year-old man has previously had retinopexy to treat a supero-temporal U tear. His vision in one eye has dropped to 6/36 over the past 2 years. At the macula there are tortuous vessels with an associated sheen.

Theme: Diseases of the vitreous I

Options

A   Anterior persistent hyerplastic primary vitreous
B   Posterior persistent hyperplastic primary vitreous
C   Amyloidosis
D   Wagner's disease
E   Stickler's syndrome
F   Familial exudative vitreoretinopathy

For each of the clinical scenarios below, select the single most likely diagnosis from the list above. Each option may be used once, more than once or not at all.

4.   This is a developmental abnormality that results from failure of the primary vitreous to regress. The hyaloid artery remains and a white vascularized fibrous membrane is present behind the lens. Associated findings include microphthalmos, shallow anterior chamber, long ciliary processes that are visible around a small lens. Leucokoria is noted at birth. There is often a cataract and anterior segment abnormality resulting in secondary narrow angle glaucoma. Amblyopia is a long-term challenge following cataract extraction.

5.   This is an autosomal dominant multisystem disorder with a mutation in the gene encoding type 11 procollagen. The vitreous cavity is empty due to vitreous liquefaction. There is associated myopia and glaucoma. There is a high incidence of retinal detachment. Generalized skeletal abnormalities including hyperextensible joints, arthritis and spondyloepiphyseal dysplaisa. Facial anomalies include flattened nasal bridge and maxillary hypoplasia. Pierre Robin malformation – micrognathia, cleft palate, glossoptosis.

6.   This is usually autosomal dominant but can be X-linked. Its characteristics are failure of temporal retina to vascularize. On fluorescein angiogram there is abrupt cessation of the retinal vasculature at the equator. There can be fibrovascular proliferation causing dragging of the macula. There is also retinal exudation and folds. It is complicated by vitreous haemorrhage, retinal detachment and cataract.

Theme: Diseases of the vitreous II

Options

A   Asteroid hyalosis
B   Synchysis scintillans
C   Jansen's disease
D   X-linked retinoschisis
E   Favre–Goldmann syndrome
F   Vitreous haemorrhage

For each of the clinical scenarios below, select the single most likely diagnosis from the list above. Each option may be used once, more than once or not at all.

7.   A 40-year-old man has had reduced vision in both eyes since he was a child. On examination he has a maculopathy that has a bicycle wheel pattern of radial striae. In the retinal periphery there are large defects in the inner retinal layer. He has recently had floaters due to vitreous haemorrhage.

8.   This condition has an autosomal dominant inheritance. There is an optically empty vitreous due to vitreous liquefaction. Fundus abnormalities include equatorial and perivascular (radial) lattice. There is a high incidence of retinal detachment.

9.   This condition presents in childhood with night blindness. It is an autosomal recessive disorder. The vitreous cavity shows syneresis but it is never empty. In the periphery there are dendritiform arborescent vessels and pigmentary changes like retinitis pigmentosa. ERG and EOG are abnormal.

Theme: Locating a retinal break I

Options
A   On the temporal side
B   At 6 o'clock
C   Above the horizontal meridien
D   Upper nasal quadrant
E   Near 12 o'clock
F   None of the above

For each of the clinical scenarios below, select the single most likely location from the list above. Each option may be used once, more than once or not at all.

10.   A shallow retinal detachment is seen in the inferior half of the retina. The subretinal fluid is slightly higher temporally. Where will the break be found?

11.   There is a bullous retinal detachment in the inferior half of the retina. Where will you find the break?

12.   There is a left small supero-temporal retinal detachment that extends from 11 o'clock to 2 o'clock. Where is the break?

Theme: Locating a retinal break II

Options
A   On the temporal side
B   At 6 o'clock
C   Above the horizontal meridien
D   Upper nasal quadrant
E   Near 12 o'clock
F   None of the above

For each of the clinical scenarios below, select the single most likely location from the list above. Each option may be used once, more than once or not at all.

13.   There is an inferior retinal detachment with fluid levels at the same height nasally and temporally. Where would you expect to find the break?

14.   There is a retinal detachment with the subretinal fluid extending around the optic disc and the upper temporal retina. Where is the break?

15.   A subtotal retinal detachment is seen with a superior wedge of attached retina. Where is the break?

Theme: Surgical treatment of the retina I

Options
A   Retinopexy and prophylactic treatment of lattice
B   Pars plana vitrectomy and fluid–gas exchange
C   Pars plana vitrectomy and encircling buckle
D   Vitrectomy and internal limiting membrane peel and fluid–gas exchange
E   Vitrectomy and membrane peel
F   Retinopexy

For each of the clinical scenarios below, select the single most suitable treatment from the list above. Each option may be used once, more than once or not at all.

16.   A 45-year-old myopic woman attends casualty with floaters in her left eye. On examination you see a Weiss ring, a superotemporal small U tear surrounded by shallow subretinal fluid. There are no other tears, holes or a retinal detachment. There are areas of peripheral lattice degeneration.

17.   A 55-year-old man with metamorphopsia is being assessed during the preoperative ward round. He has a visual acuity of 6/24, an idiopathic epiretinal membrane, a pseudohole and macular oedema confirmed on OCT. Which of the above would be the most appropriate for him?

18.   A 45-year-old man is assessed on the preoperative ward round. His vision is 6/36, he has a Weiss ring and a macula hole that is 400 µm in diameter.

Theme: Surgical treatment of the retina II

Options
A   Vitrectomy and removal of lens fragment
B   Vitrectomy and delamination
C   Vitrectomy and silicone oil
D   Pneumatic retinopexy
E   Vitrectomy and SF6
F   Vitrectomy, cryotherapy and SF6

For each of the clinical scenarios below, select the single most suitable treatment from the list above. Each option may be used once, more than once or not at all.

19.   A 60-year-old has a giant retinal tear exceeding three clock hours temporally in his left eye.

20.   A diabetic with treated proliferative diabetic retinopathy has tractional bands along the temporal vascular arcades and encroaching the macula.

21.   A 60-year-old has undergone a complicated cataract extraction that resulted in a small lens fragment being displaced into the posterior vitreous cavity. On day one postop. there is minimal anterior chamber activity.

Theme: Differential of retinal detachment

Options
A   Degenerative retinoschisis
B   Choroidal detachment
C   Uveal effusion syndrome
D   Congenital retinoschisis
E   Exudative retinal detachment
F   Bullous retinal detachment

For each of the clinical scenarios below, select the single most likely differential diagnosis from the list above. Each option may be used once, more than once or not at all.

22. A young hyperopic patient presents with a fluctuating gradual reduction in vision over a few weeks. There is no obvious retinal abnormality. Fluorescein angiography shows a leopard spot pattern abnormality. B-scan shows anterior choroidal detachment and thickening of the ciliary body.

23. A hyperopic patient referred by an optician, with bilateral absolute superonasal field defects. On examination there is no reduction in vision. There is bilateral inferotemporal inner retinal elevation and sheathing of retinal vessels. The elevated area is dome shaped with a smooth surface. There is marked cystoid degeneration of the retina. Examination of the vitreous is unremarkable.

24. A myopic patient presents complaining of misty inferior field of vision. On examination there is pigment in the vitreous, there is a Weiss ring and and a U tear superiorly with an associated shallow retinal elevation that is convex in shape.

Theme: Vitreous haemorrhage

Options
A   Terson's syndrome
B   Proliferative diabetic retinopathy
C   Age-related macular degeneration
D   Sickle cell disease
E   Eale's disease
F   Von Hippel–Lindau syndrome

For each of the clinical scenarios below, select the single most likely diagnosis from the list above. Each option may be used once, more than once or not at all.

25. A young man is referred to casualty following a head injury where he sustained a subarachnoid haemorrhage. On examination this man has preretinal haemorrhages and vitreous haemorrhages bilaterally on fundoscopy.

26. A 25-year-old man has bilateral obliterative periphlebitis in the retinal periphery. He has peripheral retinal neovascularization and vitreous haemorrhage. He is positive on a tuberculin hypersensitivity test.

27. An Afro-Carribbean man complains of sudden blurring of vision in one eye. On examination he has vitreous haemorrhage, tractional bands and a retinal detachment in that eye. The view is hazy. In the other eye he has mid-peripheral black spicules on fundoscopy, intraretinal and subretinal haemorrhages. There are sea-fan-shaped retinal neovascularization and sclerosed peripheral vessels.

Theme: Therapeutic options

Options
A   Intravitreal triamcinolone
B   Vitrectomy and removal of posterior hyaloid membrane
C   Gangciclovir implant
D   Pars plana vitrectomy, silicone oil, laser and buckle
E   Vitrectomy
F   None of the above

For each of the clinical scenarios below, select the single most suitable treatment from the list above. Each option may be used once, more than once or not at all.

28.   A 25-year-old has bilateral peripheral retinal detachments and posterior segment inflammation following a recent viral illness. He is on intravenous acyclovir and systemic steroids.

29.   An intravenous drug user presents to casualty with gradual reduction in vision. His vision is 6/60. There are white puffballs in the vitreous and there are multiple foci of infiltration in the retina at the posterior pole. The vitreous is hazy.

30.   A patient with chronic intermediate uveitis has had orbital floor injections of steroid to treat macular oedema with little response.

Chapter 8

Strabismus – EMQs

- This chapter consists of 30 extended matching questions.
- Questions consist of a theme, a list of options, an instruction and a variable number of clinical situations.
- For each of the clinical situations, you should choose the **single most likely option** according to the instruction.
- It is possible for one option to be the answer to more than one of the clinical situations.

Theme: Esotropias I

Options
A Infantile esotropia
B Primary constant accommodative esotropia
C Primary fully accommodative esotropia
D Primary convergence excess esotropia
E Primary intermittent near esotropia
F Primary intermittent cyclic esotropia

For each of the clinical scenarios below, select the single most likely diagnosis from the list above. Each option may be used once, more than once or not at all.

1. A 6-year-old girl's mother notices she has a squint when she looks closely at things. Her sister has a squint too. She is a moderate hypermetrope. She is amblyopic in the squinting eye but has good vision in her other eye. Binocular vision is normal for distance but reduced for near. She has a marked esotropia for near and an esophoria for distance. Her AC:A ratio is 7:1.

2. A 4-month-old baby boy's mother brings him in to casualty as she has noticed his left and sometimes his right eye turning inwards towards his nose. On examination he has good vision in both eyes. He cross-fixates. He also has bilateral inferior oblique overaction. There is no DVD or latent nystagmus. Refraction hypermetropia not greater than is expected for his age.

3. A 3-year-old is followed up in clinic. She wears convex glasses. She is given full refractive correction and wears a patch over her right eye. Her left eye has small convergent squint for near and distance with her glasses on. This squint is larger without her glasses on.

Theme: Exotropias I

Options
A   Primary constant exotropia
B   Primary intermittent exotropia for near
C   Primary intermittent distance exotropia (true)
D   Primary intermittent distance exotropia (simulated)
E   Sensory exotropia
F   Consecutive exotropia

4. A 60-year-old man had a right central retinal vein occlusion 2 years ago and he now has a right painful blind eye due to rubeotic glaucoma. He has a right exotropia.

5. A 21-year-old is 6/6 in both eyes. On cover test she has exophoria with good recovery for near. She has good binocular single vision for near. For distance she has an exotropia and poor binocular single vision. When a +3 D lens is placed in front of one eye she is exotropic for near. Her AC:A ratio is 7:1.

6. A 19-year-old presents with a left exotropia. His mother says he used to have this when he was younger but would only become apparent when he was tired or daydreaming, now it is there all the time. He is amblyopic in that eye. On examination the exotropia is 40 dioptres for both near and distance.

Theme: Exotropias II

Options
A   Duane's type 2
B   Internuclear ophthalmoplegia
C   Third nerve palsy
D   Sensory exotropia
E   Consecutive exotropia
F   Convergence insufficiency

7.   A 55-year-old diabetic woman attends casualty complaining of painful diplopia. On examination there is aniscoria. The right pupil is 3 mm larger than the left pupil. There is a right ptosis and weakness of right elevation and adduction. The left eye is normal.

8.   A 25-year-old woman has a left unilateral adduction weakness. In the right eye there is an abducting nystagmus. She has a skew deviation and left hypertropia. She has an associated left exotropia.

9.   On examination a 5-year-old boy's right eye has a limitation of adduction greater than abduction. Narrowing of the palpebral fissure and retraction on adduction and widening of the palpebral fissure on abduction. He has a left face turn.

Theme: Esotropias II

Options
A   Duane's type 1
B   Strabismus fixus
C   Heavy eye syndrome
D   Nystagmus blockage syndrome
E   Duane's type 3
F   Mobius syndrome

For each of the clinical scenarios below, select the single most likely diagnosis from the list above. Each option may be used once, more than once or not at all.

10.   A 3-month-old baby has a variable angle esotropia that becomes larger when fixating on an object. She has a face turn depending on which adducting eye she is using for fixation. She has an abducting nystagmus in either eye that dampens on adduction. She requires bilateral medial rectus recession and treatment of any amblyopia.

11.   A baby who is 1 month old has a large angle esotropia. Bilateral abduction weakness. Alternating face turn depending on which eye is being used to take up fixation. He has poor lid closure, and mask-like facies. The mother complains that he also has difficulty swallowing milk. In addition he is deaf. Under general anaesthetic he has a positive forced duction test and requires botulinum toxin A to medial rectus. You refer him to the paeditricians for systemic examination.

12.   A 6-year-old has an esophoria in primary position, right limitation of abduction greater than adduction. Narrowing of the palpebral fissure and retraction on adduction. Widening of the palpebral fissure on abduction. He has a right face turn. Convergence is intact.

Theme: Strabismus and systemic conditions

Options
A   Graves' disease
B   Myasthenia gravis
C   Wildervanck syndrome
D   Klippel–Feil syndrome
E   Multiple sclerosis
F   Pineal gland tumour

For each of the clinical scenarios below, select the single most likely diagnosis from the list above. Each option may be used once, more than once or not at all.

13.   A 32-year-old man presents to casualty with a 1-week history of headache. On examination he has limitation of upward eye movement, lid retraction, convergence-retraction nystagmus, skew deviation and light-near dissociation.

14.   A 10-year-old boy has a rare condition that has resulted in fusion of the second to fourth cervical spines, instability, scoliosis and Duane's syndrome.

15.   A 37-year-old woman has been admitted for intravenous immuno-globulin therapy. She has been complaining of severe difficulty in breathing. Generalized feeling of weakness in her arms and legs, started to develop difficulty swallowing and talking. The neurologists have asked for an ophthalmology opinion because she is now also complaining of diplopia and droopy lids.

Theme: Vertical strabismus

Options
A   Left fourth nerve palsy
B   Dissociated vertical deviation
C   A-pattern deviation
D   Primary inferior oblique overaction
E   Primary superior oblique overaction
F   Right fourth nerve palsy

For each of the clinical scenarios below, select the single most likely diagnosis from the list above. Each option may be used once, more than once or not at all.

16.   A 20-year-old man has a craniofacial dysostoses. There is no vertical deviation in primary position. There is bilateral depression on adduction. There is no contralateral inferior rectus weakness or ipsilateral inferior oblique weakness. There is a coexistent A-pattern.

17.   A middle-aged man has suffered a head injury after being thrown off his motorbike. He now complains of vertical diplopia. He has a head tilt towards the left, a face turn to the left and a slight chin depression. He has a positive Bielchowsky test. The most predominant finding is an inferior oblique overaction.

18.   A mother brings in her 25-year-old son as she has noticed his right eye drifting upwards. She is concerned as he had surgery as a child. He is unaware that this happens. On examination there is a slow updrift of the non-fixing eye followed by a slow recovery. It is worse in the left eye. There is no increase in elevation on adduction or abduction.

Theme: Surgical management of neurogenic palsies

Options
A   Fourth nerve palsy
B   Partially recovered sixth nerve palsy
C   Unrecovered sixth nerve palsy
D   Total third nerve palsy
E   Partial/partially recovered third nerve palsy
F   None of the above

For each of the clinical scenarios below, select the single most likely diagnosis from the list above. Each option may be used once, more than once or not at all.

19.   A 60-year-old with hypertension, diabetes and atherosclerosis developed a left esotropia 6 months ago, which was worse when looking towards the left. The esotropia is greater for distance than near. The angle of deviation has not changed between 6 and 12 months after onset. Trial with botulinum toxin to the medial rectus results in full abduction. A medial rectus recession and lateral rectus resection with adjustables is planned.

20.   A 45-year-old with microvascular palsy now 9 months later has a vertical diplopia which is worse on upgaze. He has an inferior oblique overaction with minimal superior oblique underaction. There is 14 D of vertical deviation. An inferior oblique disinsertion is planned.

21.   A 55-year-old woman with a right hypotropia requires a 12- to 15-mm lateral rectus recession on hang back and a 10-mm medial rectus resection. Each horizontal muscle is supraplaced. Stay sutures are placed transconjunctivally through the superior and inferior recti, through the tarsal plate out through the skin, and then tied tight to place the eyes in adduction and the sutures are then tied over bolsters. The stay sutures and bolsters are removed after 6 weeks.

Theme: Managing esodeviations

Options
A   Bifocals
B   Bilateral medial rectus recession
C   Unilateral medial rectus recession and lateral rectus resection
D   Orthoptic exercises
E   Cycloplegic refraction with full hypermetropic correction
F   Unilateral patching

For each of the clinical scenarios below, select the single most suitable management plan from the list above. Each option may be used once, more than once or not at all.

22.   A 3-year-old wears convex glasses. She has an intermittent esotropia, occurring when she is tired at the end of the day. Her visual acuity is 6/6 in both eyes. With her glasses she has an esophoria for near and distance and without her glasses she has a marked esotropia for near accommodative target (straight to a light target) and for distance. She has good binocular single vision with her glasses on and a normal AC:A ratio. She is not amblyopic.

23.   A 4-year-old has a squint that her mother notices is more obvious when she is looking closely at things. She is a hypermetrope. On examination she has visual acuity of 6/6 in both eyes. On cover test she has a moderate squint for a near target, esophoria for a light target. At distance she is esophoric with good recovery. Her binocular function is reduced for near but full in the distance. She has an AC:A ratio of 8:1.

24.   A 7-year-old has an intermittent esodeviation. On examination he is a hypermetrope. On cover test he is esotropic for both a near and light target. He is esophoric for distance. The near angle is quite large. AC:A ratio is normal. There is no amblyopia.

Theme: Managing exodeviations

Options
A   Bilateral medial rectus recession
B   Unilateral medial rectus resection and lateral rectus recession
C   Unilateral lateral rectus recession and medial rectus resection
D   Bilateral lateral rectus recession
E   Unilateral medial rectus resection
F   Bilateral medial rectus resection

For each of the clinical scenarios below, select the single most suitable procedure from the list above. Each option may be used once, more than once or not at all.

25.   A 2-year-old has had an exotropia since she was a few months old. It is a large angle alternating exotropia present for near and distance. There is no binocular function present. She has no refractive error. She has Crouzon's syndrome.

26.   A 19-year-old has noticed his left eye drifting outwards more than before. He finds himself closing one eye in the bright light. On examination he has an exotropia for distance and an exophoria for near. There is a 20 D difference. He describes he has panoramic vision. He does not wear glasses. He has a normal AC:A ratio. Orthoptic exercises are no longer helping. There is a marked increase in his deviation compared to previous measurements.

27.   A 30-year-old complains of headache and asthenopic symptoms after working on the computer for a given period of time. On examination visual acuities in both eyes is 6/6 corrected. He is a myope and wears glasses with base in prisms. He is intermittently exotropic for near with associated diplopia. He is exophoric for distance. The difference between the near and distance angle is 15 D. He has poor binocular function with poor convergence. There is some lateral incomitance.

Theme: Surgical procedures

Options
A   Knapp
B   Fell's modification of Harada Ito
C   Inverse Knapp
D   Jensen's
E   Schilinger's
F   Hummelscheim's

For each of the surgical procedures described below, select the single most likely name from the list above. Each option may be used once, more than once or not at all.

28.   The lateral rectus and medial rectus are moved to the border of inferior rectus to aid depression. Useful in inferior rectus palsy.

29.   In order to increase the intorsional function of the superior oblique without affecting the depressing or abducting actions, the anterior half of the superior oblique tendon is moved along the equator of the globe towards the superior border of the lateral rectus. This is useful in bilateral superior oblique palsies.

30.   The entire superior rectus and inferior rectus are moved to the insertion of the lateral rectus. This is useful in unrecovered sixth nerve palsies where botulinum toxin has no effect.

Chapter 9

Paediatric Ophthalmology – EMQs

- This chapter consists of 30 extended matching questions.
- Questions consist of a theme, a list of options, an instruction and a variable number of clinical situations.
- For each of the clinical situations, you should choose the **single most likely option** according to the instruction.
- It is possible for one option to be the answer to more than one of the clinical situations.

Chapter 9: Paediatric Ophthalmology EMQs

Theme: Electrophysiology I

Options
A   X-linked retinoschisis
B   Functional visual loss
C   Leber's amaurosis
D   Rod-cone dystrophy
E   Macular dystrophy
F   Rod-only dystrophy

For each of the clinical scenarios below, select the single most likely diagnosis from the list above. Each option may be used once, more than once or not at all.

1. A 6-month-old girl is referred by paediatricians. She has nystagmus and her parents feel she can't see very well. They also complain that she tends to rub her eyes a lot. She has been investigated by the paediatricians and is systemically well. There is no relevant family history. Her fundi are healthy on indirect ophthalmoscopy but you note that her pupillary light reflexes are very slow. On cycloplegic refraction she is slightly hypermetropic. She has had electrophysiology tests and on flash-ERG there was no measurable cone response to 30 Hz, white flash and red flash stimuli. The most probable diagnosis is . . . ?

2. An 8-month old boy attends the paediatric clinic. Vision is recorded as poor by the orthoptists. There is no ocular deviation. Pupillary reactions are normal and fundus examination is unremarkable. He has been examined by the paediatricians, who have ordered more investigations as he has problems with feeding and recently some epileptic fits. You have the results of electrophysiology. A 30-Hz flicker has elicited only minimal response and there was no response to red flash stimulus. Examination in the dark shows a very low amplitude b-wave. What is the diagnosis?

3. A 10-year-old boy has been referred from eye casualty to the paediatric ophthalmology clinic. He has seen the optician recently who is concerned as visual acuity in his left eye has deteriorated dramatically since last year. His refraction has not changed. Left visual acuity is 1/60 and right visual acuity is 6/5. Ocular examination is unremarkable. He has had electrophysiology tests. Flash ERG responses are normal. In pattern-reversal VEPs the positive component has a latency of 100 ms. This remains the same for various check sizes. The diagnosis is . . . ?

Theme: Electrophysiology II

Options
A   Congenital stationary night blindness
B   Delayed visual maturation
C   Stargardt's disease
D   X-linked retinoschisis
E   Functional visual loss
F   Albinism

For each of the clinical scenarios below, select the single most likely diagnosis from the list above. Each option may be used once, more than once or not at all.

4. A boy of 8 presents with reduced vision 6/9 and 6/18 in the right and left eye respectively. He had a history of squint. In the ERG bright stimuli generated normal a-waves but subnormal b-waves. Lower intensity stimuli generated no measurable b-waves. Fundal examination revealed abnormal findings and cystoid foveal spaces. The most likely diagnosis is ...?

5. A 3-year-old child presents with reduced vision and nystagmus. The fundi show slight hypopigmentation and the choroidal vasculature is prominent. You are ordering flash VEPs to see whether you will find hemispheric asymmetry to monocular stimulation. You are thinking of a diagnosis of ...?

6. An infant is examined at 2 and 6 months of age. There are concerns about his vision. He appears to have poor fixation and following for his age. Ocular examination is normal and the paediatricians have ruled out any systemic disorders. Neuroimaging is normal. Flash VEPS are performed at 2 and 6 months. There is a positive component to both VEPs, however peak latencies are prolonged and outside normal limits when age-matched. Peak latencies appear to shorten following subsequent visits and the child's visual acuity is improving. You are suspecting a case of ...?

Theme: Infectious ocular disease of childhood I

Options
A   Endophthalmitis
B   Herpes simplex
C   Rubella
D   Congenital toxoplasmosis
E   CMV
F   Congenital syphilis

For each of the clinical scenarios below, select the single most likely diagnosis from the list above. Each option may be used once, more than once or not at all.

7. The paediatric SpR asks you to examine a newborn girl. On examination you notice that the cornea is slightly cloudy and small. On dilated fundoscopy you cannot get a clear view of the retina but you can just about see some diffuse retinal pigment epithelial changes mainly at the posterior pole. You read in the SCBU notes that there is a congenital heart defect diagnosed on ultrasound and hepatosplenomegaly. They have also arranged an ENT review. The mother says it was generally a normal pregnancy apart from a short duration rash and fever that she suffered at the beginning. Top of your differential diagnosis would be ...?

8. Again you are examining a newborn. The paediatricians inform you that a CT scan has shown intracranial calcification around the ventricles and hydrocephalus. The baby has also suffered seizures and fever. Liver is enlarged. On examination anterior segments are quiet. In the right fundus there is a large excavated scar at the macula. You suspect a diagnosis of ...?

9. You are asked to examine a critically ill 3-year-old girl. She had been treated by her GP for the past few days for otitis media but deteriorated rapidly and is now showing signs of meningitis. She has been admitted to the paediatric ITU and has developed a very red, injected left eye. You see her urgently as you need to exclude ...?

Theme: Infectious ocular disease of childhood II

Options
A Coxsackie conjunctivitis
B Vernal keratoconjunctivitis
C Membranous conjunctivitis
D Chlamydial conjunctivitis
E Epidemic keratoconjunctivitis
F Parinaud's oculoglandular syndrome

For each of the clinical scenarios below, select the single most likely diagnosis from the list above. Each option may be used once, more than once or not at all.

10. A 12-year-old boy has been treated with systemic penicillin in the paediatric ward. He has developed a fever, cough and arthralgia and painful maculopapular and vesicular lesions in his arms, his face around his mouth and his eyelids. He also has severely injected and chemotic conjunctiva bilaterally with a characteristic appearance.

11. In the Anterior Segment clinic you are examining a 14-year-old boy with keratoconus. He has been stable so far and with good visual acuity when wearing his rigid gas permeable contact lenses. He complains that in the past few weeks he has been suffering with increasing itchiness, epiphora and intense foreign body sensation bilaterally. There are large papillae on examination of the superior tarsal conjunctiva and mucous discharge. There are limbal follicles and mild punctate corneal staining. There is an area of irregular epithelium on the superior cornea.

12. A GP refers a 3-week-old baby with bilateral sticky eyes. There is significant lid swelling, chemosis and mucopurulent discharge. It started a week after birth. You take conjunctival swabs, STD history from the mother and refer to a paediatrician.

Theme: Diseases of the conjunctiva and cornea

Options
A   Xeroderma pigmentosa
B   Goldenhaar's syndrome
C   Sturge–Weber syndrome
D   Louis–Bar syndrome
E   Lymphohaemangioma
F   Wyburn–Mason syndrome

For each of the clinical scenarios below, select the single most likely diagnosis from the list above. Each option may be used once, more than once or not at all.

13. A 4-year-old Asian girl attends the children's clinic. She has a long-standing left conjunctivitis. Her skin has multiple telangiectasic lesions and shows diffuse pigmentation. She had excision of basal cell carcinomas in the past.

14. An 18-month-old boy attends the clinic. He has obvious signs of mental handicap and growth regression. He is frequently in hospital as he has an immune deficiency syndrome. Examination of the anterior segment shows some tortuous vessels in the temporal conjunctiva of the right eye.

15. A 3-year-old girl attends her follow-up in the paediatric clinic. She has a history of multiple subconjunctival haemorrhages in the right eye and she has a large fleshy red lesion arising from the lateral conjunctiva. On close observation there is a mixture of clear and blood-filled cysts in this lesion.

Theme: Cornea

Options
A   Cornea plana
B   Keratoconus
C   Keratoglobus
D   Peter's anomaly
E   Corneal dermoid
F   CHED (congenital hereditary endothelial dystrophy)

For each of the clinical scenarios below, select the single most likely diagnosis from the list above. Each option may be used once, more than once or not at all.

16.   A 16-week-old girl is brought to the clinic by her parents. They have noticed opacities of the cornea more in the right than the left eye. There is a stromal opacity on the visual axis of both eyes. The right cornea is definitely smaller than the left. The baby had surgery to correct a cleft lip and palate shortly after birth. You also think you can see a cataract in the right eye.

17.   A 2-week-old baby is referred to your team by the paediatricians. There are bilateral marked cloudy oedematous corneas. Her father has had bilateral penetrating keratoplasties in the past.

18.   A 13-year-old boy with Down's syndrome has been referred by the optician because his refraction has been changed significantly in the past year with increasing myopic astigmatism. You suspect . . . .

Theme: Lens disorders

Options
A   Wilson's syndrome
B   Lowe's syndrome
C   Nance–Horan syndrome
D   Galactossaemia
E   Hallerman–Streiff syndrome
F   Weill–Marchesani syndrome

For each of the clinical scenarios below, select the single most likely diagnosis from the list above. Each option may be used once, more than once or not at all.

19. You are examining a 3-week-old baby. She appears to have an abnormal red reflex due to opacities in the lens. There is an 'oil-droplet' appearance of the red reflex. She has jaundice and the paediatricians are concerned because of failure to thrive.

20. A 3-year-old boy attends the clinic referred by the paediatricians. The parents are concerned because of deterioration in his visual acuity. On examination the right eye appears to be slightly microphthalmic. There are lens opacities bilaterally. He has a typical facial appearance with small chin, frontal prominence, thin nose with thin-veined skin and progeric appearance.

21. A 4-year-old girl has been referred by a paediatrician. She has developmental delay and intermittent aminoaciduria. They are concerned about her vision. On retro-illumination she appears to have multiple punctate lens opacities.

Theme: Retina

Options
A   Coat's disease
B   FEVR (familial exudative vitreo-retinopathy)
C   Incontinentia pigmenti
D   Toxocariasis
E   Stickler's syndrome
F   Retinal capillary haemangioma

For each of the clinical scenarios below, select the single most likely diagnosis from the list above. Each option may be used once, more than once or not at all.

22.   In the paediatric clinic you are asked to examine a 4-year-old boy. He has been referred by his optician due to a left divergent squint. The right eye is healthy with no refractive error and a visual acuity of 6/5. The left eye is divergent with a visual acuity of 6/36. Fundal examination shows large areas of telangiectasic vessels and retinal exudates peripherally.

23.   A 2-year-old girl with ectodermal dysplasia attends the clinic. She has vesicular skin lesions. On examination of the fundi there are areas of scattered retinal fibrosis and the right eye has an inferotemporal tractional retinal detachment and longstanding macular oedema. She has had photocoagulation treatment in the past.

24.   A 2-year-old attends the clinic with her mother. They are both highly myopic, with broad nasal bridge and wear hearing aids. The mother has had multiple vitreo-retinal procedures. The child appears to have very syneretic vitreous and perivascular retinal pigmentary changes. There are areas of peripheral chorioretinal degeneration. You follow her up closely.

Theme: Skin lesions

Options
A   Haemangioma of the eyelid
B   Port-wine stain
C   Keratoacanthoma
D   Strawberry naevus
E   Plexiform neurofibroma
F   Pyogenic granuloma

For each of the clinical scenarios below, select the single most likely diagnosis from the list above. Each option may be used once, more than once or not at all.

25.   You are called to examine a newborn baby because the paediatricians have noticed a well-demarcated, subcutaneous pink patch involving the left side of face over the baby's forehead and cheek. The overlying skin is slightly swollen. The baby has also had a few fits.

26.   A 10-year-old girl has been referred by her GP to the paediatric ophthalmology clinic. The GP is concerned about unilateral ptosis. There is a lesion on the left upper lid giving the lid an S-shaped pattern. Your consultant asks you to examine her iris and optic nerve. You note that she has been under the paediatricians for a long time.

27.   The paediatricians have referred a 12-month-old girl because of a red-purple lesion under the right eyebrow. The father has noticed it for sometime but it has increased in size over the past 4 months. The mother says she is not too bothered by its appearance at the moment but relatives and friends comment on it especially when the baby is crying. She shows you the child's right arm which has a similar small red spot.

Theme: Lid abnormalities

Options
A   Congenital myogenic ptosis
B   Muscular dystrophy
C   Blepharophimosis
D   Marcus Gunn jaw winking syndrome
E   Congenital Horner's syndrome
F   Neurogenic ptosis

For each of the clinical scenarios below, select the single most likely diagnosis from the list above. Each option may be used once, more than once or not at all.

28.   You are examining a 3-week-old baby. He has a slightly ptotic eyelid on the left side. The left palpebral aperture is much lower than the right. Levator function is about 5 mm. The mother mentions that the ptosis improves slightly when the baby is lying flat and breastfeeding.

29.   A 2-year-old child attends the clinic. He has moderate bilateral ptosis. Levator function is 7 mm on the right and 6 mm on the left side. You note he has a larger fold on the lower lid compared to the upper lid. There is a mild ectropion on the lower lid of the left eye. There is definitely an abnormal nasal bridge and the medial canthi look slightly displaced.

30.   A 3-year-old child has been referred by his GP. He has a droopy eyelid on the right side and a small convergent squint that he controls by wearing his hypermetropic prescription. Visual acuities are 6/6 in the right eye and 6/5 in the left eye. Parents say they had no major concerns up to this date as the ptosis is not affecting his vision. On slit-lamp examination you notice the iris is a slightly lighter colour on the right side.

Chapter 10

Neuro-ophthalmology – EMQs

- This chapter consists of 21 extended matching questions.
- Questions consist of a theme, a list of options, an instruction and a variable number of clinical situations.
- For each of the clinical situations, you should choose the **single most likely option** according to the instruction.
- It is possible for one option to be the answer to more than one of the clinical situations.

Theme: Pupils I – mydriasis

Options
A   Iatrogenic
B   Adie's syndrome
C   Third nerve palsy
D   Syphilis
E   Physical anisocoria
F   None of the above

For each of the clinical scenarios below, select the single most likely diagnosis from the list above. Each option may be used once, more than once or not at all.

1. A 65-year-old diabetic woman presents with painless diplopia. She has a mild ptosis, exotropia, mid-dilated pupil. The anisocoria is greater in light and reduced in the dark. There is no RAPD.

2. A woman in her mid-30s presents with a 1-week history of left painless dilated pupil. She has no RAPD. In the left there is a sluggish direct and indirect response to light. Re-dilatation is slow. There is poor accommodative response in the left eye. On slit-lamp examination of the left iris there is a superotemporal segment of iris palsy. The anisocoria is more obvious in the light. A pharmacological test was used to confirm the diagnosis. Deep tendon reflexes were intact.

3. A 70-year-old has a dilated pupil. He had a complicated cataract operation that resulted in a posterior capsular tear. One quadrant of soft lens matter was displaced into the posterior segment. He needed a vitrectomy. He had persistent postoperative inflammation and raised intraocular pressure. He required a trabeculectomy with mitomycin C.

Theme: Pupils II – miosis

Options

A   Physiological anisocoria
B   Brainstem stroke
C   Argyll Robertson
D   Aberrant regeneration following third nerve palsy
E   Pancoast's tumour
F   Syringomyelia

For each of the clinical scenarios below, select the single most likely diagnosis from the list above. Each option may be used once, more than once or not at all.

4. An elderly woman presents to casualty with a 2-day history of a 'funny feeling' around her right eye. On examination she has a right miosis, ptosis and apparent enophthalmos. Fundus examination is normal and fields are full. There is no other focal neurology. Chest X-ray shows a right apical opacity. She is referred to the respiratory physicians.

5. An elderly lady in a wheelchair. She has shooting pains in her legs. Examining her pupils, both her pupils are irregular and constricted, she has poor direct and indirect light responses but a good response to accommodation.

6. A 40-year-old male has unilateral miosis, a mild ptosis, normal light and near pupillary reactions. He has longstanding sexual dysfunction. He has diffuse muscle atrophy of his hands. He has loss of pain and temperature sensations, but light touch, vibration and proprioception are intact. A previous MRI revealed a fluid-filled cavity within the spinal cord.

Theme: Multiple cranial nerve palsies

Options
A   Cavernous sinus syndrome
B   Foville's syndrome
C   Lateral medullary syndrome
D   Subarachnoid space syndrome
E   Cerebellopontine angle tumour
F   Millard–Gubler syndrome

For each of the clinical scenarios below, select the single most likely diagnosis from the list above. Each option may be used once, more than once or not at all.

7. A 70-year-old man as a result of a cerebrovascular accident has developed neuralgia in the distribution of the Vth cranial nerve, nystagmus with the fast phase towards the left, dysarthria and dsyphagia and right miosis, ptosis and apparent enophthalmos. On sensory examination he has reduced pain and temperature sensation on the right side of his face and reduced pain and temperature sensation on the left leg. He has an intention tremor, hypotonia and ataxic gait.

8. A young woman with neurofibromatosis-2 presents with nystagmus, reduced corneal sensation and right lateral rectus paresis and right lower motor neuron facial nerve palsy. She also has a left hemiplegia.

9. A 65-year-old woman has shingles in the ophthalmic branch of the Vth cranial nerve. She also complains of diplopia. On examination she has IIIrd, IVth and VIth nerve palsies. Fundal examination is normal.

Theme: Headache

Options

A   Raeder's syndrome
B   Giant cell arteritis
C   Cluster headache
D   Basilar artery migraine
E   Pseudotumour cerebri
F   Ocular migraine

For each of the clinical scenarios below, select the single most likely diagnosis from the list above. Each option may be used once, more than once or not at all.

10.   A 65-year-old Caucasian woman attends casualty with severe pain around her right eye. She has a history of polymyalgia rheumatica. She complains of pain on chewing food that occurs after a period of time, the temporal artery is tender on palpation, it is non-pulsatile and thickened. She also complains of a reduction in vision and on examination she has a swollen disc.

11.   An 18-year-old overweight girl has acne. She has been prescribed oral tetracycline, which she has been using for 8 months. She has had a generalized headache for one month. She describes transient visual obscurations. She has bilateral swollen optic discs. She has bilateral enlarged blind spots. Further investigations reveal raised intracranial pressure and normal cerebrospinal fluid composition.

12.   A 55-year-old man presents with pain in the ophthalmic branch of the Vth cranial nerve. He has a ptosis, miosis and an apparent enophathlmos. Investigation excludes a parasellar mass. There are no other cranial nerves involved. This condition is thought to be due to migrainous dilatation of the internal carotid artery with compression of the V1 and sympathetic plexus in the middle cranial fossa.

Theme: Optic disc pallor

Options
A 'Optic nerve glioma'
B Optic nerve meningioma
C Tobacco-alcohol amblyopia
D Leber's hereditary optic neuropathy
E Arsenicosis
F De Morsier's syndrome

For each of the clinical scenarios below, select the single most likely diagnosis from the list above. Each option may be used once, more than once or not at all.

13. An 18-year-old man presents with bilateral, sequential, acute reduction in vision. His vision is 6/36 in both eyes. On fundoscopy he has bilateral swollen discs with abnormal vessels, which look like telangiectasia. He has a central scotoma. He is advised not to smoke or drink alcohol and advised regarding a healthy diet.

14. A woman of 20 is registered blind. She is short in stature, has hemifacial atrophy and congenital nystagmus. She is known to have a septo-optic dysplasia and on fundoscopy there is a double ring sign. She is also hypothyroid and has diabetes insipidus. She has not started menstruating yet.

15. A 4-year-old girl was brought in to casualty by her mother, because of rapid onset proptosis and loss of vision. MRI scan shows double intensity tubular thickening and kinking of the orbital nerve. She is referred to a neurologist to exclude neurofibromatosis. A multi-disciplinary meeting is arranged to decide if she should be treated surgically or using radiotherapy or chemotherapy.

Theme: Phakomatoses

Options
A   Neurofibromatosis 1
B   Neurofibromatosis 2
C   Tuberous sclerosis
D   Von Hippel–Lindau disease
E   Sturge–Weber syndrome
F   Ataxia telangiectasia

For each of the clinical scenarios below, select the single most likely diagnosis from the list above. Each option may be used once, more than once or not at all.

16.   This condition is seen in 1 in 50 000. It is an autosomal dominant trait and the gene is located on chromosome 22. Patients usually have less than six café-lait spots. Ocular examination reveals bilateral posterior subcapsular cataracts and combined hamartoma of RPE and the retina. Bilateral vestibular schwannomas are the hallmark of this syndrome, causing tinnitus, hearing loss and vertigo. Other tumours include schwannomas of cranial nerve, peripheral nerves and spinal nerves, meningiomas of optic nerve sheath, intracranial and intraspinal, gliomas and ependymomas.

17.   The hereditary pattern of this condition is unknown. Patients have facial angioma from birth. It is usually unilateral, follows the distribution of the ophthalmic, maxillary and mandibular branches of the trigeminal nerve. This is associated with hemi-hypertrophy of the face. 60% of patients have secondary glaucoma that is difficult to control. Some patients have choroidal haemangiomas with associated retinal detachment. There are also angiomas of the conjunctiva and sclera. The central nervous system has leptomeningeal haemangioma located between the pia and arachnoid often located over the parieto-occipital cortex. The underlying cortex is maldeveloped and hypoplastic. Calcium deposition in the blood vessels shown on CT scan looks like a tram-track. 75% of patients have epileptic seizures. Others are hemiplegic and have a homonymous hemianopia.

18.   This condition is known as angiomatosis of the retina and cerebellum. It occurs in 1 in 36 000. It is inherited as autosomal dominant with incomplete penetrance. There are no cutaneous lesions. The main ocular lesion is a retinal haemangioblastoma. It can be treated with photocoagulation or cryotherapy. In the central nervous system haemangioblastomas are located in cerebellum, spinal cord and brainstem. In the third decade of life patients present with raised intracranial pressure, renal cell carcinomas, phaeochromocytoma and benign cysts of the kidneys, pancreas, liver and epididymis.

Theme: Facial nerve disorders

Options
A   Crocodile tears
B   Bell's palsy
C   Meige's syndrome
D   Intrinsic pontine tumour
E   Ramsay Hunt syndrome
F   Cerebellopontine angle tumour

For each of the clinical scenarios below, select the single most likely diagnosis from the list above. Each option may be used once, more than once or not at all.

19.   A 30-year-old woman with hearing loss. On examination she has vesicles in her external auditory meatus. This infection results in inflammation of the internal auditory meatus. She has drooping of the corner of her mouth on the right side, right cheek paralysis and right upper lid ptosis. She complains of a watery eye. There is no other associated neurological deficit.

20.   Several months after recovering from lower motor neuron facial nerve palsy a 50-year-old man complains of watery eye after chewing food. This occurs due to abberant regeneration of parasympathetic fibres stimulating tears and salivation.

21.   A 65-year-old woman has bilateral episodic, involuntary contraction of the orbicularis oculi and this is associated with involuntary spasm of the lower facial musculature.

Chapter 11

General Medicine – EMQs

- This chapter consists of 18 extended matching questions.
- Questions consist of a theme, a list of options, an instruction and a variable number of clinical situations.
- For each of the clinical situations, you should choose the **single most likely option** according to the instruction.
- It is possible for one option to be the answer to more than one of the clinical situations.

Chapter 11: General Medicine EMQs

Theme: Medical emergencies I

Options
A   Cardiorespiratory arrest
B   Hyperglycaemic hyperosmolar non-ketotoic acidosis (HONK)
C   Diabetic ketoacidosis
D   Type 1 anaphylactic shock
E   Acute myocardial infarction
F   Unstable angina

For each of the emergency scenarios below, select the single most likely diagnosis from the list above. Each option may be used once, more than once or not at all.

1. An elderly woman sitting in the outpatient waiting area complains of chest pain. Her companion says that she has had previous heart surgery. An immediate ECG shows ST depression, and inverted T waves in the lateral leads. The pulse rate is 70 per minute. The airway is clear and she is breathing. You place a high flow oxygen mask over her face, give her 300 mg aspirin and sublingual GTN. You urgently speak to the on-call cardiologist who arranges to review her.

2. A type 1 diabetic gives a 2- to 3-day history of feeling unwell. He has recently had a chest infection. He says he feels thirsty and complains of urinary frequency and on examination he is dehydrated and is vomiting and has sweet-smelling breath. He has high serum glucose levels, blood gases reveal acidosis, he has a high white cell count and is hyponatraemic. Urine dipstick test contributes to making a diagnosis. He requires immediate intravenous fluids (0.9% saline) and 10 units of intravenous insulin. An insulin sliding scale is set up and potassium replacement started.

3. A patient collapses in the waiting area. Her blood pressure is 90/40 mmHg. Her skin has a yellow discoloration and she is having difficulty breathing. You place a high flow oxygen mask over her mouth. Lay her flat on her back with feet up. Administer intravenous 0.5 ml adrenaline (epinephrine) 1:1000, intravenous prednisolone 200 mg and intravenous piriton 10 mg. You contact the medical registrar on call to review her.

Theme: Treating medical emergencies

Options
A   Cardiogenic shock
B   Acute severe asthma
C   Pulmonary embolism
D   Status epilepticus
E   Myxoedema coma
F   Thyrotoxic storm

For each of the emergency scenarios below, select the single most likely diagnosis from the list above. Each option may be used once, more than once or not at all.

4.   A collapsed patient is placed in the recovery position, an oral airway is inserted and treated with 100% oxygen, intravenous lorazepam 4 mg and bloods for U&Es, LFTs, FBC, glucose and calcium.

5.   Initial treatment of this emergency involves sitting the patient up, administering high dose oxygen, 5 mg salbutamol nebulized wth oxygen, 200 mg intravenous hydrocortisone. An urgent chest X-ray is requested.

6.   This emergency is treated initially with intravenous saline, sedation with chlorpromazine, propranolol and possibly digoxin to slow down the tachycardia, carbimazole and Lugol's solution and prednisolone. Treatment of any underlying infection is important.

Theme: Brainstem syndromes involving cranial nerves

Options
A   Weber's syndrome
B   Claude's syndrome
C   Benedikt's syndrome
D   Nothnagel's syndrome
E   Wallenburg's syndrome
F   Parinaud's syndrome

For each of the syndromes described below, select the single most likely diagnosis from the list above. Each option may be used once, more than once or not at all.

7.   Site of lesion is tegmentum of medulla. It affects the Vth, IXth, Xth and XIth cranial nerves. It also involves the lateral spinothalamic tracts, descending pupillomotor fibres, spinocerebellar and olivo-cerebellar tracts. Presentation is with ipsilateral Horner's, cerebellar ataxia, ipsilateral Vth, IXth, Xth and XIth lesions. There is contralateral loss of pain and temperature. This is caused by occlusion of vertebral or posterior inferior cerebellar artery.

8.   This syndrome occurs with a lesion in the tectum of the midbrain. Presents with a unilateral or bilateral third nerve palsy. It also involves the superior cerebellar peduncles, causing paralysis of gaze and cerebellar ataxia. It occurs due to a tumour.

9.   This occurs due to a vascular occlusion, aneurysm or tumour of the midbrain it involves the third cranial nerve nuclei and corticospinal tract resulting in oculomotor palsy and crossed hemiplegia.

Theme: Movement disorders

Options
A   Parkinson's disease
B   Steele–Richardson syndrome
C   Huntingdon's chorea
D   Wilson's disease
E   Shy–Drager syndrome
F   Sytemic lupus erythematosus

For each of the conditions described below, select the single most likely diagnosis from the list above. Each option may be used once, more than once or not at all.

10.   These patients have orthostatic hypotension, degeneration of the extrapyramidal tracts, basal ganglia and dorsal nucleus of the vagus. These patients fail to increase their secretion of neurotransmitter during standing and exercise.

11.   This is an inherited autosomal recessive abnormality. Results in deficiency of caeruloplasmin. It results in toxic accumulation of the brain, liver and other organs. Half of patients present with hepatic involvement. Neurological manifestations are always accompanied by Kayser–Fleischer rings and include resting and intention tremor, spasticity, rigidity, drooling, dysphagia, dysarthria. Psychiatric disturbances include schizophrenia and manic-depressive psychosis.

12.   A 50-year-old man has seborrheic skin changes, reduced blink reflex and a downgaze palsy. Saccadic eye movements are unaffected. There is no resting tremor. He is experiencing recurrent falls.

Theme: Spinal cord disorders

Options
A   Brown–Sequard syndrome
B   Progressive muscular atrophy
C   Amyotrophic lateral sclerosis
D   Progressive bulbar palsy
E   Friedreich's ataxia
F   Subacute combined degeneration of the spinal cord

For each of the clinical scenarios below, select the single most likely diagnosis from the list above. Each option may be used once, more than once or not at all.

13. A 12-year-old previously healthy girl develops problems with walking. Her mother says she staggers when walking and has difficulty in standing. She also suffers from clumsiness with her hands and an intention tremor. She has developed scanning speech. All these changes are due to changes in the dorsal root ganglion, cerebellar and spinocerebellar tracts. The limbs are also considerably weak. On examination there is a nystagmus, kyphoscoliosis, pes cavus and atrophy and contracture of the foot muscles.

14. This occurs due to vitamin B_{12} deficiency. The brain, optic nerve and peripheral nerves may also be involved. There is also associated pernicious anaemia. A patient will first notice tingling, paraesthesia of distal limbs which can be distressing. As the illness progresses the gait becomes unsteady and movements of the legs become stiff and awkward. The nervous system involvement is characteristically symmetrical. The spinal cord involvement is of the posterior and lateral columns. Loss of vibration sense in the legs is pronounced. Motor signs include loss of power and spasticity in the legs. Reflexes can be increased or absent. Sensory signs are uncommon.

15. A 60-year-old presents with muscular atrophy and hyperreflexia combined. The weakness and muscular wasting is asymmetrical and widespread. Classically it presents in the small muscles of the hand. Eventually dysarthria and impairment of swallowing develop. The ocular nuclei tend to be spared. There is exaggeration of tendon reflexes. Progression is rapid with death from respiratory failure within 2–5 years.

Theme: Peripheral sensory neuropathy

Options
A   Diabetes mellitus
B   Amyloidosis
C   Vitamin B$_{12}$ deficiency
D   Leprosy
E   Carcinomatous neuropathy
F   Uraemic neuropathy

For each of the clinical scenarios below, select the single most likely diagnosis from the list above. Each option may be used once, more than once or not at all.

16.   This disorder is characterized by extracellular deposits of abnormal beta-pleated, degradation resistant proteins. This protein stains positive with Congo red and shows green birefringence in polarized light. There are two disease forms: (i) local and (ii) systemic. It can be primary which in 50% is associated with myeloma. It can be secondary to chronic infections such as TB, chronic inflammations such as rheumatoid arthritis and neoplasias. It can affect the kidneys, spleen and liver and cause congestive cardiac failure.

17.   This is a distal sensorimotor polyneuropathy caused by toxins associated with secondary demyelination. It can also be associated with mononeuropathy at compression sites. It results in paraesthesia and increaesd pain sensation. Weakness of lower extremities and atrophy follow sensory symptoms, then as the disease progresses symptoms move proximally to involve the upper extremities. Patients also complain of muscle cramps and restless leg syndrome. It is also associated wth autonomic dysfunction resulting in postural hypotension. Rapid respiratory failure has also been reported.

18.   This disease is the only mycobacterium known to infect nervous tissue. Results in anaesthetic, non-itchy skin lesions, diminution to complete loss of sensation, paraesthesia in distributon of affected nerves and neuralgic pain when the nerve head is struck or stretched. The tuberculous form is affected by sensory loss than the lepromatous form.

Answers

Chapter 1: Adnexal and Orbit Answers

Theme: Lid lesions I

1. **C**
2. **F**
3. **B**

Papillomas can be confused with pedunculated seborrhoeic keratosis but they tend to be constricted at the base and are more common in elderly patients.

Cutaneous horns are equal in females and males and more common in older patients. They are raised with white stalky appearance and very hyperkeratotic surface.

Molluscum contagiosum association with HIV/immunocompromised patients. Also can be spread by skin-to-skin contact.

Syringomas appear as multiple lesions in lower lids of women. They appear in puberty. May be familial. May also be found in face, axilla, upper chest and vulva.

Keratoacanthoma should be differentiated from squamous cell carcinoma and the only way is histopathology after excision.

Theme: Lids

4. **C**
5. **E** – Blepharitis is a bilateral condition. Recurrent chalazion or unilateral blepharitis in an elderly patient must alert you to sebaceous adenocarcinoma.
6. **A**

An **apocrine hydrosystoma** is a cystic lesion arising from the glands of Moll on the eyelid margin. Usually translucent and transilluminates.

Theme: Lid lesions II

7. **B** – Subcutaneous and present at birth. Gradually the overlying skin becomes oedematous and harsh. Port-wine stain darkens with age. In 5% of cases associated with Sturge–Weber syndrome. Ipsilateral angiomas of the meninges and brain cause epileptic fits, hemiparesis, etc. 30% of ipsilateral facial angiomas, especially if upper eyelid involvement, are associated with glaucoma.
8. **E** – Associated with neurofibromatosis-1.
9. **D** – Strawberry naevus tends to resolve with age. 75% resolve by the age of 4. Presentation at 6–12 months. Remember deep lesions can present with proptosis. Rhabdomyosarcoma must be excluded (only with biopsy)! If risk of amblyopia, consider intralesion steroids but remember risks (skin depigmentation, skin necrosis, risk CRAO, etc.).

Theme: Neoplasms of the lid I

10. **C** – Lentigo maligna is an intraepidermal neoplasm. It is premalignant. It can give rise to lentigo maligna melanoma.
11. **E**
12. **D** – 90% of malignant lid tumours are BCCs. Medial canthus BCCs are aggressive and difficult to manage. Neglected ones can spread in the orbit and cause extraocular muscle restriction. Generally they do not metastasize to regional lymph nodes. Multiple BCCs can be found in younger patients with basal cell carcinoma syndrome.

Keratoacanthoma is a benign lesion but needs to be differentiated from SCC. 1:1000 cases of actinic keratosis will give rise to SCC.

Theme: Neoplasms of the lid II

13. **E** – If you suspect sebaceous gland carcinoma alert the pathologist for fat stains, otherwise SCC may be misdiagnosed histologically.
14. **A** – Tumour thickness is the most important predictor of prognosis. If <0.76 mm it has 93.2% 8-year survival rate. If >3.60 mm deep it has 33.3% 8-year survival rate. There are two classic histological classifications: Clark (anatomical level of involvement) and Breslow (tumour thickness).
15. **D**

Theme: Treating lid lesions

16. **B** – For very elderly and debilitated patients who are not fit for surgery and major reconstruction, cryotherapy is preferable. It is a single session treatment. There is a 10% recurrence rate and it should be avoided in patients with darkly pigmented skin! (Risks: hypertrophic scar, depigmentation, ectropion, long healing time, lid notch.) It is also preferable in cases where the tumour is involving the punctum, as radiotherapy is contraindicated for medial canthus lesions (damage to puncta, dry eye, conjunctival keratinization, loss of lashes, skin necrosis, cicatricial changes).
17. **D** – A medial canthus BCC would most likely need major reconstruction. When it involves the caruncle there is a possibility it may have involved deeper orbital tissues. In order to determine clearance of the base of the lesion a two-stage procedure with fast paraffin or Moh's micrographic technique is necessary.
18. **C** – If following excision of a lower lid neoplasm, the remaining defect is 25% or less it can be closed directly. In older patients with significant lid laxity even lid defects of 25–50% can be closed directly. In younger patients where the lids and skin may be quite tight, in order to avoid tension on the wound we will have to consider performing canthotomy and cantholysis.

Theme: Surgical procedures

19. A
20. F
21. C

Tenzel (semicircular) flap is indicated for repair of lower lid defects that involve up to 70% of the eyelid and where the fellow eye has poor vision. A Hughes (upper lid tarsoconjunctival flap) is a better solution provided that the fellow eye has good visual acuity as after a Hughes, the affected eye will remain closed for about 6–8 weeks according to the healing process!

Burrow's triangles refer only to a detail in surgical technique (and they are not a method of reconstruction). They are relaxing incisions at the edges of a defect.

A glabellar flap is used for large medial canthal region defects. However it leaves the patient with forehead scarring and the eyebrows appear to be closer postoperatively. It works best for elderly patients with a lot of tissue laxity.

Theme: Surgical interventions

22. **A** – The Cutler–Beard reconstruction is best left to the hands of an experienced oculoplastic surgeon. This method is indicated for extensive (100%) upper lid defects. Remember to refer the patient with an extensive upper lid SCC. A cartilage graft may need to be used for tarsal reconstruction and the skin defect is repaired as well.
23. **F** – The O-Z flap is indicated for circular defects with excess skin where stretching of the skin would not result in ectropion postoperatively.
24. **E** – NB: never 'laissez-faire' an upper lid defect involving the lid margin.

Theme: Eyelid and canalicular trauma

25. **C** – If the medial canthus is avulsed, which is more common in dog bites, check the canalicular system. The anterior and posterior limbs of the medial canthus need to be repaired. Metronidazole orally is necessary to protect from infection from anaerobic bacteria. Tetanus status needs to be checked as well.
26. **A** – Lacerations of the levator aponeurosis can sometimes heal on their own if less than half of its width is damaged. If there is major trauma to the levator, aim to repair initially all the other eyelid structures and the lid margin (primary repair) and you can plan repair of the levator (traumatic ptosis surgery) at a second stage when the degree of ptosis can be assessed more accurately. The **exception** to this is children at risk of occlusion amblyopia! Such severe injuries to children are rare but if the ptosis and the swelling do not resolve quickly they may need a temporary brow suspension to prevent amblyopia.
27. **B**

Theme: Canalicular procedures

28. **A**
29. **C**
30. **B**

US ophthalmologists tend to repair all canalicular lacerations with intubation. Evidence shows that there is not a significant difference in the outcomes. Generally if both canaliculi are severed there should be a discussion with the patient regarding intubation. Care should be taken not to injure an intact canaliculus while trying to intubate the injured one. If direct repair with marsupialization is undertaken especially for the lower canaliculus, warn the patient about the possibility of a secondary procedure in the future. Lacrimal sac injuries need primary DCR with intubation.

Theme: Cicatricial lid malpositions

31. **A**
32. **B**
33. **C**

All these are surgical solutions for cicatricial ectropion. Khunt–Symanovsky and LCS are preferred procedures in cases of involutional ectropion. Lazy-T is for medial (involutional) ectropion.

Theme: Eyelid malpositions

34. **B**
35. **E** – Congenital distichiasis is present at birth and refers to a second row of lashes growing posterior to the normal eyelashes. Risk of corneal scarring.
36. **F** – Epiblepharon is congenital and refers to override of the pretarsal muscle and skin. The cilia have a vertical position. The lid margin however has a normal position. It rarely causes corneal complications and children are generally asymptomatic.

Theme: Entropion I

37. **F** – Tarsal dissection +/− MMG is indicated in many cases of cicatricial entropion.
38. **A** – Anterior lamellar repositioning +/− grey line split is the most common way of repairing mild to moderate upper lid entropion. Other methods are very subspecialized. Consider everting sutures only for very mild lower lid entropia and possibly in elderly patients that cannot tolerate long operating times. Be careful when tightening to avoid punctal ectropion.
39. **E** – Jones' (plication of lower lid retractors) is indicated in recurrences. Other methods for lower lid entropion correction are Wies procedure and Quickert's preocedure. In Quickert's, the Wies surgical technique is combined with horizontal lid shortening.

Theme: Entropion II

40. **B** – This is a central ectropion with no canthal laxity. A pentagon excision with direct closure offers a good solution, however when there is excess skin, a Khunt–Symanovsky procedure (pentagon + lower lid blepharoplasty) offers a better result.
41. **C**
42. **D** – Tarsoconjunctival diamond excision for punctal ectropion with no horizontal laxity. If there is horizontal laxity and the medial canthus is intact, a lazy-T procedure is preferable. If the medial canthal tendon is lax, then consider plication of the anterior and posterior limbs of the medial canthal tendon, or if medial canthal laxity is severe consider medial canthal resection.

Theme: Adnexal clinic I

43. **B** – The patient possibly had a temporary tarsorrhaphy and she obviously has a gold weight on her upper lid (paralytic ectropion).
44. **A** – The patient has a pressure pad on his pre-auricular area, therefore a skin graft must have been harvested at the time of the operation from that area. Skin grafts are used to correct combined horizontal and vertical skin shortage as in cicatricial ectropion.
45. **E** – Large cysts and chemosis pull the lid down causing mechanical ectropion.

Theme: Ptosis I

46. **D**
47. **C** – Blepharophimosis syndrome: ptosis moderate to severe (symmetrical or slightly asymmetrical), telecanthus, epicanthus inversus, hypertelorism, lower lid ectropion, nasal bridge hypoplasia. Autosomal dominant inheritance.
48. **E**

Theme: Ptosis II

49. **A** – Check acetylcholine receptor antibodies, thyroid function. Refer to neurology for possible tensilon test and single fibre EMG. If symptoms are severe and diagnostic refer urgently to physicians as respiratory compromise could be life threatening!
50. **D** – Autosomal dominant inheritance generally. Presenile cataracts (daughter has already had cataract extractions). Ptosis, difficulty in release of grip, mournful expression due to bilateral facial weakness. Slurred speech from involvement of pharyngeal muscles. Frontal baldness in males. May have cardiac anomalies.
51. **F** – This is pseudoptosis due to left enophthalmos.

Theme: Ptosis III

52. **A** – In simple congenital ptosis the levator is dysgenetic and as a result the muscle has a problem both when contracting and relaxing. (Ptotic eyelid remains higher than normal eyelid at downgaze.)

53. **E** – Kearns–Sayre syndrome: pigmentary retinopathy and heart block (causes sudden death). Mitochondrial myopathy. Also cerebellar ataxia, muscle weakness, neurosensory deafness and delayed puberty. Usually diagnosed before the age of 20 years.

54. **D** – Gene on chromosome 12. Oculopharyngeal dystrophy: autosomal dominant inheritance pattern. Ptosis + weakness of pharyngeal muscles.

Theme: Adnexal clinic II

55. **C** – Blepharochalasis, a type of angioneurotic oedema. Usually unilateral and affects females in their teens or 20s. Recurrent episodes of eyelid inflammation. Skin appears stretched and may have the appearance of dermatochalasis as seen in older patients. May be accompanied by lacrimal gland prolapse.

56. **A** – All of these are brow lift procedures.

57. **B**

Theme: Ptosis surgery

58. **F** – Fasanella–Servat or tarsomullerectomy is indicated for very mild ptosis (about 2 mm) with good levator function.

59. **D**

60. **C** – Severe ptosis with poor levator function (LF < 4 mm) requires brow suspension (bilateral in children). For adults the suspensory material is autogenous fascia lata which is harvested from the thigh. This cannot be used for children under the age of four. In these cases non-autogenous materials can be used such as Mersilene mesh, Supramid, silicone cords. Surgically the Crawford technique is used for autogenous material and the Fox pentagon when non-autologous material is used. Levator resection and aponeurosis advancement are indicated in myogenic or neurogenic ptosis with moderate or good levator function (LF > 5 mm).

Theme: Postoperative management of ptosis surgery

61. **E** – Marked overcorrection: release bands as soon as possible. Undercorrection: if significant immediately postoperation tighten bands as soon as possible. Consider redo surgery.

62. **F** – Overcorrection – unacceptably high upper lid: immediate lowering. Overcorrection – mild: option as described in B. Significant undercorrection: immediate repeat surgery. Lash ptosis: skin crease reformation or if skin crease is present anterior lamellar repositioning.

63. **C** – Repeat surgery. If possible try to use autogenous fascia lata (result more longstanding).

Theme: Congenital eyelid anomalies

64. **F** – Ankyloblepharon can be congenital or acquired. It is acquired in cases of OCP, Stevens–Johnson, chemical burns. Failure of the eyelids to separate during embryonic development is congenital.

65. **B** – Epiblepharon needs to be differentiated from congenital entropion. Pull the excess skin back (override of the pretarsal muscle and skin) and you will find that the lid margin has a normal position.

66. **D** – Lid colobomas are full thickness lid defects (abnormal embryonic development). Upper lid colobomas are usually isolated. However lower lid colobomas are associated with cleft facial syndromes. Surgical repair has excellent prognosis and is necessary to protect the cornea.

Theme: Lacrimal apparatus

67. **E**

68. **D** – If the mass is below the medial canthal tendon it is most likely a dacryocystocele. If the mass is located above the medial canthal tendon you need to think about the possibility of an encephalocele or haemangioma.

69. **C** – Lacrimal fistula: rare, congenital but can present at any age. One-third of these are related to lacrimal system stenosis.

Theme: Lacrimal system surgery

70. **C** – In patients with progressive scarring and inflammatory diseases such as OCP, it is wise to avoid canalicular tubing as this may exacerbate the inflammatory process and contribute further to dry eye problems.

71. **A** – This is a typical NLD obstruction.

72. **B** – A soft stop indicates obstruction in the canalicular system. Reflux through the upper canaliculus indicates obstruction in the common canaliculus. Regurgitation from the lower canaliculus would indicate stenosis of the same canaliculus. With common canalicular obstruction a DCG is helpful to show the site of obstruction of the common canaliclus (lateral or medial obstruction = slight variation in surgical technique). A Lester Jones tube is indicated in cases where there is single canalicular obstruction where <8 mm of canaliculus is patent. If >8 mm canaliculus is patent a cDCR will suffice.

Theme: Orbit

73. **B** – (phycomycosis = mucormycosis). Fungi spread to the orbit from the adjacent sinuses or nose. Common in poorly controlled diabetics, immunocompromised patients, malignancies, after chemotherapy, etc.

74. **E**

75. **F**

Theme: Lid lesions I

76. **C**
77. **F**
78. **A**

Theme: Orbital lesions I

79. **C**
80. **A**
81. **F**

Theme: Orbital lesions II

82. **E**
83. **A**
84. **B** – low-flow fistula, Doppler is diagnostic as it will show reversal of flow in the superior ophthalmic vein.

Theme: Orbital lesions III

85. **B**
86. **C**
87. **E**

Theme: Orbit

88. **A**
89. **B**
90. **D**

Theme: Management of orbital disease

91. **D** – Routine orbital referral if inactive inflammation, if there is significant proptosis or even if IOPs are high.
92. **C** – If good response to systemic steroids refer early for low dose radiotherapy.
93. **B** – Some orbital specialists agree that radiotherapy is contraindicated in diabetic patients as there is a risk of developing diabetic retinopathy.

Theme: Treating orbital lesions

94. **C** – This is a case of orbital myositis (muscle tendon is involved on CT). Consider oral steroids if no response to oral NSAIDs.
95. **D** – Never commence oral steroids if you suspect orbital infiltration. Refer urgently to orbital specialist for biopsy!
96. **E** – This is the one case where you would need to decompress without waiting to refer to an orbital surgeon.

Theme: Lacrimal gland

97. **B** – 'Salmon-patch' appearance is typical for lymphomas.
98. **C** – Sarcoidosis needs to be excluded in this case, but the presentation with progressive unilateral proptosis and the CT scan point to the diagnosis. Note that adenomas of the lacrimal gland do not cause bony erosion and do not present with calcification. Prognosis is excellent if excised completely. If left they can give rise to malignancy.
99. **F** – Dacryops. Clinical picture different than dacryoadenitis – note 'bursts of lacrimation'. Remember the 'S-shaped ptosis' in dacryoadenitis.

Theme: Management of corneal exposure

100. **A** – Usually lubricants and taping the eyelid down at night are sufficient. However if there is significant corneal exposure, a temporary lateral tarsorrhaphy needs to be considered.
101. **D** – Lateral canthal sling has good results for repair of paralytic ectropion. The medial canthal tendon needs to be assessed. A medial canthoplasty is usually enough, but if there is marked laxity of the MC tendon, a medial wedge resection would give a better outcome.
102. **B** – The gold weight is obvious on a patient's upper eyelid. There are other ways of lowering the upper lid such as Muller's muscle excision or recession or recession of both Muller's and the levator. However the gold weight gives a more satisfactory blinking.
Lester Jones tube can be used for cases of severe epiphora.

Theme: Corneal exposure

103. **A** – Botox-induced ptosis offers temporary closure of the eye without subjecting the patient to a surgical procedure. Warn the patient the eye will be closed for about 6 weeks but that can be variable!
104. **B** – The skin is very tight in this case and he probably had some skin loss at the time of the injury.
105. **C** – This is subspecialized surgery and should be carried out by oculoplastic surgeons. In this case both the skin and lid retractors are tight.

Theme: Congenital orbital malformations

106. **C**
107. **B**
108. **A**

Hypertelorism is increased distance between the two eyes due to excess bone in the medial orbital walls. May be found on its own but is also associated with other craniofacial abnormalities such as clefts, encephaloceles, etc.
In **Apert's syndrome** there is lateral positioning of the orbits and lateral canthal malposition. Amblyopia, strabismus and optic atrophy can occur. Associated with heart, lung and renal problems.

Theme: Socket

109. **B** – volume deficiency is compensated with a larger prosthesis and, as a result, the prosthesis becomes unstable, the lower lid becomes lax, there is no inferior fornix.
110. **A** – volume deficiency (PESS): enophthalmos, deep upper sulcus, ptosis.
111. **C** – lining deficiency: congenital (anophthalmos, microphthalmos) or acquired (trauma, burns, inflammation).

Theme: Orbital trauma

112. **B** – Orbital floor fractures require repair only when there is persistent functional diplopia or enophthalmos. Generally it is considered appropriate for this to be repaired within 2 weeks of the time of injury. In children, however, there is high possibility of entrapment of the inferior rectus and that should be operated withn 24–48 hours to prevent muscle ischaemia and longstanding motility problems.
113. **D** – Medial wall fractures do not require repair unless the medial rectus is entrapped causing diplopia.
114. **F** – An orbital roof fracture may have CNS complications and is repaired via craniotomy, so it needs to be referred to neurosugeons!

Generally be aware: small fractures have higher chances of causing entrapment than large fractures!

Chapter 2: Cornea and External Eye Disease Answers

Theme: Ectasias

1. **C**
2. **B**
3. **E**

Posterior keratoconus: thinning results from an increase in posterior corneal curvature. It can be diffuse or localized. In the diffuse form the cornea remains clear. In the focal form there is a central or paracentral area of excavation associated with variable amounts of stromal scarring. It is usually unilateral. It is usually developmental. It may be confused with Peter's anomaly but unlike Peter's anomaly the corneal endothelium and Descemet's membrane is not absent or thinned.

Keractasia is a rare congenital usually unilateral condition due to intrauterine keratitis and perforation. It presents with severe corneal opacification and protruberance beyond the eyelids.

Theme: Conjunctival disorders

4. **F**
5. **B**
6. **D**

Theme: Acute conjunctivitis

7. **A** – Corneal perforation can occur rapidly following a corneal ulcer. Gonococcal conjunctivitis should be treated urgently and followed up frequently. Referral to GU clinic for an STD screen and contact tracing is essential.
8. **C** – Pharyngoconjunctival fever. Incubation period is 5–7 days and fever can last up to 14 days.
9. **E** – Atopic people can suffer from bilateral HSV-1 keratoconjunctivitis.

Theme: Chronic conjunctivitis

10. **E**
11. **A** – In a patient with multiple molluscum HIV should always be considered. It is easy to miss small lesions hidden among eyelashes. Careful lid examination is essential in those with chronic ocular pruritis with follicular conjunctivitis.
12. **C** – What is the WHO classification for trachoma?

Theme: Cicatrizing conjunctivitis

13. **A** – Linear IgA disease is very rare indeed. Occurs in young children or adults typically above the age of 60 but can occur in younger patients as in this case. Due to IgA deposition in, eg, basement membrane of dermal–epidermal junction and other tissues including conjunctiva. A histological diagnosis is made by immunofluorescence.

14. **B** – Ocular cicatricial pemphogoid:
Stage 1 = Subepithelial fibrosis
Stage 2 = Forniceal shortening
Stage 3 = Symblepharon formation
Stage 4 = Ankyloblepharon and surface keratinization

15. **C**

Theme: Herpes simplex virus

16. **A** – The exact pathogenesis of endotheliitis is unknown. There are three forms: disciform, linear and diffuse. It appears that it is an immunological reaction at the level of the endothelium. The role of live virus has been speculated. Resolution is achieved with topical corticosteroids.

17. **B** – Stromal keratitis is a common recurrent manifestation of HSV keratitis occurring in 20% of ocular HSV. Inflammation is thought to be triggered by retained viral antigen within the stroma that in turn triggers an antigen–antibody–complement cascade.

18. **D** – Herpetic Eye Disease Study (HEDS) II.

Theme: Interstitial keratitis

19. **D** – Cogan's syndrome is associated with Wegener's granulomatosis, polyarteritis nodosa, rheumatoid arthritis, Crohn's disease, relapsing polychondritis and systemic vasculitis. In the late stages vascularization and ghost vessels occur. Initially could be misdiagnosed as a viral keratitis. If left untreated profound deafness can develop. Treatment involves systemic immunosuppression.

20. **A** – Onchocerciasis is a parasitic disease caused by the nematode *Onchocerca volvulus*. It is often referred to as river blindness. Occurs in West, Central and East Africa and parts of South America.

21. **F**

Theme: Therapeutic indications for contact lens wear

22. **B** – Soft bandage contact lens interrupts the mechanical factors existing between the superior tarsus and bulbar conjunctiva. It is useful in patients with filaments.

23. **F**

24. **D**

Theme: Complications of contact lens wear

25. C
26. B
27. A

Theme: Secondary causes of corneal astigmatism

28. E
29. B
30. C

Theme: Corneal graft surgery

31. **C** – Fuch's endothelial dystrophy.
32. **D** – Herpes simplex virus keratitis.
33. **F** – Large diameter and eccentric (pellucid margin degeneration).

Theme: Corneal opacity and scarring

34. C
35. **F** – A published series has shown that 76–100% of patients on 200–800 mg/day have verticillata. Verticillata does not affect vision. Rarely irreversible vision loss occurs from amiodarone optic neuropathy.
36. D

Theme: Corneal disease associated with systemic diseases

37. F
38. D
39. C

Theme: Corneal dystrophies

40. D
41. E
42. B

Theme: Ocular causes of peripheral ulcerative keratitis

43. E
44. F
45. B

Theme: Systemic causes of peripheral ulcerative keratitis

46. B
47. C
48. E

Theme: Microbial keratitis

49. **F**
50. **B**
51. **C**

Theme: Treatment options

52. **E**
53. **A**
54. **D**

Theme: Systemic treatment options

55. **A** – OCP; more acutely inflamed OCP requires pulsed prednisolone or second-line immunosuppression.
56. **B** – Scleritis due to Wegener's responds to cyclophosphamide.
57. **E**

Theme: How would you manage this?

58. **E**
59. **B** – If this fails then PTK.
60. **F** – Culture on a small plate of non-nutrient agar which will require *E. coli* overlay.

Theme: Prominent corneal nerves

61. **C**
62. **E**
63. **B**

Theme: Managing Fuch's endothelial dystrophy

64. **B**
65. **E**
66. **A**

Chapter 3: Refractive Surgery Answers

Theme: Refractive procedures

1. **C**
2. **B** – In hyperopia the cornea is made steeper by reducing the central radius of curvature to increase the optical power.
3. **A**

Theme: LASIK complications

4. **E** – Diffuse lamellar keratitis is also known as 'Sands of Sahara':
   Grade 1: Focal grey granular material; acuity not reduced
   Grade 2: Diffuse white-grey granular material; acuity not reduced
   Grade 3: Diffuse, confluent material; reduced acuity
   Grade 4: Diffuse confluent and intense central inflammation; reduced acuity.
   Treatment = irrigation beneath flap, topical steroids and daily review.
5. **F** – Flap striae:
   Grade 1: Fine parallel lines; difficult to detect; VA unaffected
   Grade 2: Fine parallel lines; obvious; reduced VA; <1 D astigmatism
   Grade 3: Large lines; reduced VA; >1 D astigmatism.
   Treatment = flap lifted and repositioned.
6. **B** – Epithelial ingrowth can vary in severity and affect visual acuity. It is associated with flap melt.

Theme: Correcting hyperopia

7. **C** – This is a variant of PRK.
8. **A**
9. **E**

Theme: Correcting myopia

10. **E** – Warn patient of presbyopia. C is also an option: the Artisan iris claw lens isn't used commonly in the UK but data have been reported from mainland Europe and the USA. A corneal procedure would be at higher risk of aggravating HSV keratitis, eg LASIK/LASEK could result in marked postoperative interface haze or even corneal perforation.
11. **D** – Intacs implantation of two ultrathin PMMA arcs of 150 degree segments to two-thirds corneal depth. This alters the corneal curvature, flattening it and thus reducing myopia.
12. **A** – Scleral sling was rarely used in the past for −18 to −22 D myopia. Donor sclera/synthetic material was used to sling around the globe.

Chapter 4: Glaucoma Answers

Theme: Acute raised intraocular pressure

1. **A**
2. **E** – Occurs as a result of pigment release from the RPE following a large retinal detachment. The raised pressure is rectified by repair of the retinal detachment.
3. **C**

Theme: What is the cause of low intraocular pressure?

4. **E**
5. **A**
6. **C**

Theme: Secondary glaucomas

7. **E**
8. **A**
9. **D**

Theme: Landmark studies

10. **A**
11. **E**
12. **A**

Theme: Surgical/laser treatment

13. **E** – Uveitic patients. A drainage tube is more likely to survive than a trabeculectomy if surgery such as a cataract extraction is required in the future.
14. **A**
15. **D** – Blacks/Asians are at higher risk of trabeculectomy failure and thus require mitomycin C.

Theme: What is the glaucoma diagnosis?

16. **B**
17. **A**
18. **F**

Theme: What is the mechanism of raised intraocular pressure?

19. **B** – Pigment dispersion syndrome.
20. **D** – Plateau iris syndrome is a form of narrow angle glaucoma.
21. **A** – Scleritis can cause anterior rotation of the ciliary body and thus a secondary narrow angle glaucoma. Treatment is high dose intravenous steroids followed later by a surgical iridectomy.

Theme: Investigating glaucoma

22. **C**
23. **A**
24. **D**

Theme: Complications of a trabeculectomy

25. **C** – Careful follow-up is required as blebitis can progress to endophthalmitis.
26. **B**
27. **F** – The site of leakage will be Siedel's positive.

Theme: Medical therapy

28. **E/F** – Always ensure the patient isn't diabetic when using glycerol.
29. **C**
30. **B** – Plateau iris.

Theme: HLA associations

1. **C**
2. **D**
3. **A**

HLA A11 – Sympathetic ophthalmitis.
HLA A29 – Bird shot chorioretinopathy (relative risk = 97%).
HLA B51 – Behçet's.
HLA B7 – Presumed ocular histoplasmosis (POHS), multiple sclerosis.
HLA B12 – Cicatricial pemphigoid.
HLA B17 – Psoriasis.
HLA B22 – Vogt–Koyanagi–Harada syndrome (VKH).
HLA B27 – Ankylosing spondylitis (relative risk = 90%), Reiter's, psoriatic arthropathy.
HLA Bw44 – Stevens–Johnson syndrome.
HLA Bw54 – Possner–Schlossmann.
HLA Drw54 – VKH.
HLA DR3 – Sjörgen's, SLE, TED, juvenile diabetes mellitus, myasthenia gravis.
HLA DR4 – Rheumatoid arthritis, juvenile diabetes mellitus.

Theme: Intermediate uveitis

4. **D** – Lyme disease is a multisytem infection caused by *Borrelia burgdorferi*, which is transmitted by the bite of Ixodidae ticks (deer is the host of the mature tick). It is common in midwest USA and sporadic in Europe. After an incubation period of 3–30 days a flu-like illness follows. The bite causes a skin lesion as described above called erythema chronicum migrans. The signs and symptoms disappear over several weeks. The second phase causes excruciating headaches, cranial nerve palsies, heart blocks, arthropathy of large joints, encephalopthy causing impaired mood, sleep and memory. In the eye it causes conjunctivitis, choroiditis, retinal oedema and papilitis. The eye signs can occur at any stage.
5. **B**
6. **A**

A thorough systemic enquiry is essential to guide you towards a diagnosis other than **idiopathic**. Investigations should really only be necessary if clinical findings or systemic enquiry makes you suspect a diagnosis other than idiopathic.
Differential of unilateral intermediate uveitis: ocular toxocariasis; peripheral retinal toxoplasmosis; Fuch's heterochromic cyclitis; amyloid infiltrate of vitreous; Coat's disease; Schwartz syndrome (uveitis and high IOP associated with retinal tear or detachment).

Theme: Uveitis

7. **E/D** – Behçets' disease.
8. **C** – Juvenile chronic anterior uveitis.
9. **A** – Bird-shot chorioretinopathy.

Theme: Inflammatory conditions of the choroid and retina

10. **B**
11. **C**
12. **E**

Krill's disease is an uncommon condition that can be either uni- or bilateral. Thought to be preceded by a viral illness. Patients present with blurring and metamorphopsia. Typical lesions are grey in the outer retina with a yellow rim. They occur in clusters of 3 or 4 and have a honeycomb appearance. Fluorescein angiography has progressive staining of the affected RPE. As a rule visual recovery is good.

Theme: Posterior uveitis

13. **B**
14. **F** – Predominantly retinal arterial occlusion but mixed artery and venous occlusion seen.
15. **C** – Predominantly retinal venous occlusion but mixed artery and venous occlusion seen.

Theme: Treatment options in uveitis

16. **D** – CMV retinitis in a patient not on HAART.
17. **A** – Eale's disease has no ocular inflammation, ie quiet eye/no cells. Differential of retinal phlebitis; sarcoid, Behçet's, TB, syphilis.
18. **B** – Intermediate uveitis (pars planitis if snowbanking present) and CMO.

Theme: Surgical interventions in uveitic eyes

19. **C** – Trabeculectomy is likely to fail.
20. **B** – This has been shown to be relatively successful in Presumed Ocular Histoplasmosis Syndrome. Unlike in AMD (type 1 membrane that has broken through only Bruch's), inflammatory membranes (type 2) are situated between the neurosensory retina and RPE (broken through both Bruch's and RPE).
21. **F** – Unmodified PMMA lenses attract cellular deposits which are more marked in uveitic eyes.

Theme: Anterior uveitis

22. **B** – HLA B27 associated with anterior uveitis can occur without any association with systemic disease. 71% of patients with recurrent unilateral anterior uveitis are HLA B27+ve.
23. **E** – Also known as glaucomacyclitic crisis. The inflammation is predominantly confined to the trabecular meshwork.
24. **C** – Reiter first described the syndrome as a triad of non-specific urethritis, conjunctivitis and arthritis.

Theme: Systemic therapy in inflammatory conditions

25. **B** – Wegener's granulomatosis and anterior scleritis responds to cyclophosphamide.
26. **F** – Ocular cicatricial pemphigoid. High dose steroid is required for highly active and rapidly progressive cases. Such cases are not common.
27. **C** – Reactivation of toxoplasmosis chorioretinitis. Major side-effect of clindamycin is pseudomembranous colitis.

Theme: Uveitis and systemic disease

28. **B**
29. **F**
30. **D**

Chapter 6: Medical Retina Answers

Theme: Clinical trials in the management of diabetic retinopathy

1. **A**
2. **C**
3. **D**

Theme: ETDRS classification of diabetic retinopathy

4. **F**
5. **C**
6. **D**

Theme: Managing diabetic retinopathy I

7. **B**
8. **D** – Panretinal photocoagulation first followed by laser to the macula.
9. **A**

Theme: Managing diabetic retinopathy II

10. **A**
11. **C** (NB: the treatment effect may only last for the duration of triamcinolone and CSME returns in 3–4 months – hence some centres don't do this.)
12. **B**

Theme: Vein occlusion

13. **F**
14. **C** (CRVO)
15. **D**

Theme: Vascular retinopathy

16. **B**

Sickle cell disease (SS) – mild ocular complications, severe systemic disease.
Sickle cell thalassaemia (Sthal) – severe ocular complications, mild systemic disease.
Sickle cell haemoglobin C disease (SC) – severe ocular complications, mild systemic disease.
Sickle cell trait – mild ocular complications, mild systemic disease.

17. **C**
18. **E**

Theme: Age-related macular degeneration

19. **A**
20. **E** (Or Ocuvite for smokers to minimize lung cancer risk.)
21. **C** (Visual acuity between 6/12 to 6/60 eligible according to NICE guidelines.)

Theme: Vitreous haemorrhage

22. **E**
23. **B** – A breakthrough bleed from a subretinal neovascular membrane can present as a vitreous haemorrhage.
24. **A**

Theme: Investigations

25. **E** – Homocysteine levels in the young are also important.
26. **B**
27. **C** – This is treated as a sickle cell crises.

Theme: Fluorescein angiogram I

28. **A**
29. **E** – Irvine–Gass doesn't occur 1 week postoperatively and the peak incidence occurs 6–10 weeks postoperatively.
30. **B**

Theme: Fluorescein angiogram II

31. **A**
32. **B**
33. **E** (Early HYPOfluorescence then late HYPERfluorescence of the yellow Dalen's Fuch's nodules.)

Theme: Hereditary retina I

34. **A**
35. **F** – This is fundus flavimaculatus, although this and Stargardt's are thought to be different spectrums of the same disease entity. Electrodiagnostics are carried out routinely at Moorfields and is used to provide prognostic information:

    ERG Pattern Type 1 = maculopathy ⎫ Non-progressive
    ERG Pattern Type 2 = maculopthy and ⎬ retinopathy
    　　　　　　　　　　　　cone dystrophy ⎭

    ERG Pattern Type 3 = maculopathy　　⎫ Progressive
    　　　　　　　　+ cone + rod dystrophy ⎭ retinopathy

36. **B**

Theme: A negative ERG

37. **B**
38. **D** – Melanoma-associated retinopathy.
39. **E**

NB: A negative ERG describes the waveform pattern when there is an absent b-wave. It is a feature of abnormal ganglion cell layer and inner retinal layer function.

Theme: Hereditary retina II

40. **E**
41. **F**
42. **D** – Usher's type 1 profound early onset deafness; type 2 less severe deafness.

Theme: Subretinal neovascular membrane

43. **D**
44. **E** – 50% have no systemic associations.
45. **B** – A normal vitreous is an important negative finding.

Theme: Acquired diseases affecting the macula

46. **D**
47. **A**
48. **C**

Theme: Clinical trials

49. **C**
50. **D**
51. **E**

Theme: Systemic diseases associated with pigmentary retinopathy – autosomal dominant

52. **A**
53. **D**
54. **E**

Charcot–Marie–Tooth: pigmentary retinopathy, degeneration of lateral horn of spinal cord, optic atrophy.
Myotonic dystrophy: proximal muscle wasting, Christmas tree cataract, retinal degeneration, pattern dystrophy, subnormal ERG.
Oculodentodigital syndrome: thin nose with hypoplastic alae, narrow nostrils, abnormality of fourth and fifth fingers, hypoplastic dental enamel, congenital cataract, colobomas.

Theme: Systemic disease associated with pigmentary retinopathy – autosomal recessive

55. **F** – Mucopolysaccharidoses.
56. **B**
57. **A**

Homocystinuria:
Fine pigmentary or cystic degeneration of the retina, marfanoid appearance, myopia, inferior subluxation or dislocation of the lens, cardiovascular abnormalities, glaucoma, mental retardation.

Mannosidosis:
Resembles Hurler's syndrome; macroglossia, flat nose, large head and ears, skeletal abnormalities, hepatosplenomegaly and storage material in the retina.

Hurler's syndrome (mucopolysaccharidoses):
Early clouding of the cornea, gargoyle facies, deafness, mental retardation, dwarfism, skeletal abnormalities, hepatosplenomegaly, optic atrophy, subnormal ERG.

Theme: Miscellaneous

58. **F**
59. **D** – Chronic carotid artery obstruction. Chronic ophthalmic artery obstruction can cause a similar picture.
60. **E**

Chapter 7: Vitreo-retinal Disorders Answers

Theme: Vitrectomy for macular diseases

1. **B** – The traction vectors are anteroposterior in vitreo-macula traction syndrome whereas in epiretinal membrane they are tangential.
2. **C**
3. **A**

Theme: Diseases of the vitreous I

4. **A** – In posterior PHPV the anterior segment is normal and the lens is clear without a retrolenticular membrane.
5. **E**
6. **F**

Theme: Diseases of the vitreous II

7. **D**
8. **C**
9. **E**

Hereditary hyaloideoretinopathies with optically empty vitreous: there is vitreous liquefaction except for a thin layer of cortical vitreous behind the lens and a whitish avascular membrane that adheres to the retina.
No systemic abnormalities –
1) Jansen's disease, high incidence of retinal detachment;
2) Wagner's disease, low incidence of retinal detachment.
Systemic abnormalities –
Stickler's syndrome; Weill–Marchesani syndrome.

Theme: Locating a retinal break I

10. **A**
11. **C**
12. **E**

Theme: Locating a retinal break II

13. **B**
14. **D**
15. **F**

Theme: Surgical treatment of the retina I

16. **F**
17. **E** – Some surgeons are known to also use an encircling band to prevent retinal detachment but there is no evidence to support this.
18. **B/D** – Use of adjuvant pharmacological agent, eg transforming growth factor beta, autologous serum or internal limiting membrane (ILM) peel remains controversial.

Theme: Surgical treatment of the retina II

19. **C**
20. **B**
21. **A** – Small pieces with no inflammation or intraocular pressure problems don't require surgical intervention.

Theme: Differential of retinal detachment

22. **C**
23. **A**
24. **F**

Theme: Vitreous haemorrhage

25. **A**
26. **E**
27. **D**

Theme: Therapeutic options

28. **D** – Acute retinal necrosis. Silicone oil is required because a single break is difficult to identify and large areas of retina are thinned and damaged and because proliferative retinopathy is common.
29. **F** – Candida endophthalmitis.
30. **A**

Theme: Esotropias I

1. **D**
2. **A** – DVD appears many months/years after onset.
3. **B**

Theme: Exotropias I

4. **E**
5. **D** – To identify whether the exotropia is true or simulated, perform two manoeuvres: (i) reduce accommodative convergence by placing a +3 D lens in front of one eye; (ii) reduce fusional convergence by occluding one eye. Both these steps increase the angle for near in simulated distance exotropia.
6. **A**

NB: A baby/young child with an exotropia should be investigated for neurological, metabolic or craniofacial abnormalities if a refractive error is excluded.

Theme: Exotropias II

7. **C** – This patient should be scanned to exclude a compressive lesion such as an aneurysm.
8. **B**
9. **A**

Theme: Esotropias II

10. **D** – The esotropia develops to enhance monocular acuity by dampening nystagmus using convergence.
11. **F**
12. **E**

Heavy eye syndrome is progressive esotropia and hypotropia in high myopes. MRI studies suggest prolapse of the globe inferonasally due to nasal shift of the superior rectus and inferior shift of the lateral rectus.

Theme: Strabismus and systemic conditions

13. **F**
14. **D**
15. **A**

Theme: Vertical strabismus

16. **E**
17. **F**
18. **B** – DVD and inferior oblique often coexist and can be difficult to differ-entiate. A DVD does not change depending on direction of gaze, whereas an inferior oblique overaction increases on adduction and is reduced on abduction.

Theme: Surgical management of neurogenic palsies

19. **B**
20. **A**
21. **D**

Theme: Managing esodeviations

22. **E** – Fully accommodative intermittent esotropia. Surgery should not be performed despite parental requests unless there is decompensation to a constant strabismus.
23. **A** – Primary intermittent accommodative esotropia of convergence excess type.
24. **B** – Intermittent non-accommodative near esotropia.

Accommodative esotropias occur because there is a high accommodative drive.
Non-accommodative esotropias occur because there is increased tone in baseline convergence.

Theme: Managing exodeviations

25. **B** – Primary constant exotropia.
26. **D** – Intermittenet true distance exotropia.
27. **E** – Intermittent exotropia for near.

Theme: Surgical procedures

28. **C**
29. **B**
30. **E** – This is effective in conjunction with botulinum toxin to the medial rectus 1 week prior to surgery. The eye is left exotropic at the end of surgery and as the toxin wears off it will move medially.

Chapter 9: Paediatric Ophthalmology Answers

Theme: Electrophysiology I

1. **C** – Leber's congenital amaurosis: autosomal recessive inheritance. Presents with blindness. Slow pupillary light reflexes, may have optic disc atrophy and pigmentary changes but fundi are generally normal initially. Nystagmus is common. Oculodigital syndrome occurs as a result of eye rubbing. Non-recordable ERG. Infants could be systemically well or have associated epilepsy, deafness and/or mental handicap.

2. **D** – In flash-ERG rod and cone responses can be separately assessed. Rod activity can be suppressed by adaptation to a low intensity white light and by using a bright flash stimulus, then the ERG response generated will be from the cones only. Low intensity flashes presented to a dark-adapted eye generate a signal from the rods. A 30-Hz flicker produces a cone response. In a dark-adapted eye a bright flash of light will produced a mixed cone-rod response. The a-wave (negative) is mainly produced by the photoreceptors and the b-wave (positive) mainly from the inner nuclear layer. Oscillatory potentials are generated by cells in the inner retina.

3. **B** – Pattern-VEP (checkerboard) is very useful. In pattern-reversal VEP the elements of the checkerboard are reversed in contrast in a periodical way. The latency and amplitude of the individual peaks are analysed. There is a positive component with a latency of 100 ms (P100). In this example, a normal ERG and normal pattern VEP point to the diagnosis of functional visual loss.

Theme: Electrophysiology II

4. **D** – In X-linked retinoschisis the inner retinal layers are affected, therefore the b-wave is subnormal or absent especially in eyes with a peripheral retinoschisis. ERG may be normal in eyes with isolated maculopathy.

5. **F** – VEP is diagnostic in albinism, as in albinos only 10–20% of fibres remain uncrossed at the chiasm (45% in normals). As a result each occipital cortex receives a monocular projection of the central visual field.

6. **B** – Full investigation of children with 'delayed visual maturation' is necessary before reaching this diagnosis, as there may be associated neurological, developmental and ocular anomalies. The VEPs however are often normal or they improve when repeated at later age.

Theme: Infectious ocular disease of childhood I

7. **C** – Ocular and systemic signs of rubella infection. Ocular: cataracts (25%), RPE changes at retina mainly at posterior pole, microphthalmos, glaucoma, cloudy cornea. Systemic signs: deafness, congenital heart defect, hepatosplenomegaly, microcephaly. History of maternal rash and fever especially at first trimester of pregnancy.

8. **D** – Congenital toxoplasmosis can also cause chorioretinits, uveitis, secondary cataracts and cerebral blindness.

9. **A** – Causes of paediatric endophthalmitis: keratitis, metastatic (meningitis, endocarditis, otitis), trauma, surgery. Remember possibility of fungal infection (candida-ill children in SCBU). Toxocara and toxoplasmosis can also present with endophthalmitis.

Herpes simplex: mother would have history of genital herpes simplex. Ocular signs: uveitis (may be necrotizing), cataract, chorioretinitis. Systemic signs: 100% skin rash, triad of encephalitis/hepatitis/pneumonitis.
CMV: rare but chorioretinitis, keratitis can affect vision permanently.
Congenital syphilis: infection is more severe after 18 weeks' gestation. Ocular signs: interstitial keratitis, uveitis/chorioretinitis, possibly salt-and-pepper retinopathy, optic atrophy. Systemic signs: rash (maculopapular), nose deformities, rhinitis, dental abnormalities, deafness.

Theme: Infectious ocular disease of childhood II

10. **C** – Causes of membranous conjunctivitis (fibrinous membrane over ocular surface and cornea): in this case Steven–Johnson and toxic epidermal necrolysis; also herpes simplex and zoster infections, *Corynebacterium diphtheriae*.

11. **B** – Typical VKC. Associated with atopy (keratoconus in this case). There is usually a history of asthma and eczema. Remember Tranta's dots, shield ulcers and vernal 'plaques'.

12. **D** – This is now becoming a more common cause of neonatal conjunctivitis as up to 12% of women have genital chlamydial disease. Ask for Giemsa stain (intracytoplasmic inclusion bodies). Now ELISA techniques are used. Remember ocular infection may be associated with systemic infection, especially pneumonitis in 10–20% cases, so need to refer to a paediatrician for systemic (erythromycin) treatment. Parents need to be counselled and treated as necessary.

Coxsackie viruses cause haemorrhagic conjunctivitis (multiple subconjunctival haemorrhages).
Epidemic keratoconjunctivitis: mainly follicular reaction – highly infectious.
Parinaud's oculoglandular syndrome: conjunctivitis and lymphadenopathy.

Theme: Diseases of the conjunctiva and cornea

13. **A** – Autosomal recessive, risk of BCCs, SCCs and malignant melanomas! Light photosensitivity.
14. **D** – Louis–Bar or ataxia-telangiectasia: autosomal recessive, immune deficiency, growth delay, telangiectasias on conjunctiva.
15. **E** – Clear and blood-filled cysts are characteristic for the diagnosis of lymphohaemangioma.

Goldenhaar's syndrome: limbal dermoid, eyelid colobomas, pre-auricular skin tags, and vertebral abnormalities.
Wyburn–Mason syndrome: intracranial and orbital vascular anomalies and racemose retinal haemangiomas.

Theme: Cornea

16. **D** – Peter's anomaly: bilateral congenital central corneal opacification. Peripheral cornea is clear. Adhesions between lens and cornea and a cataract may be present. Associated with iris abnormalities, glaucoma, microcornea, cornea plana. Peter's syndrome: cleft lip/palate, short stature, ear abnormalities. Peter's can be present in fetal alcohol syndrome.
17. **F** – CHED is present at birth. Histologically, Descemet's membrane is abnormal and endothelium is atrophic. As a result the whole cornea is oedematous and thick with a bluish-white hue. May improve spontaneously with time but if risk of amblyopia requires PK at an early stage.
18. **B** – Later onset than previous conditions, usually >10 years old.

Keratoglobus is a rare bilateral condition with thinning of the whole cornea. Present at birth, no progression. Risk of corneal perforation.
Cornea plana: cornea with curvature 20–40 D. Associated with glaucoma, aniridia, colobomas, congenital cataracts, microphthalmos. Usually high hypermetropia.

Theme: Lens disorders

19. **D** – Jaundice and failure to thrive are characteristic. The child is usually systemically unwell. 'Oil-droplet' appearance of red reflex. Early changes are reversible with dietary control.
20. **E** – 85% have microphthalmic eyes.
21. **B** – X-linked. Males more severely affected with microphthalmos, congenital glaucoma. Prognosis is poor.

Wilson's disease: sunflower cataract.
Nance–Horan syndrome: X-linked disorder. Males more severely affected with congenital dense cataracts, iris abnormalities, dental abnormalities and prominent ears.

Theme: Retina

22. **A** – This is Coat's disease. FEVR is usually bilateral and more severe.
23. **C** – Associated with ectodermal dysplasia, vesicular skin lesions. Lethal in males (X-linked dominant).
24. **E**

Theme: Skin lesions

25. **B** – Port-wine stains darken with age. They are subcutaneous and present at birth. Gradually the overlying skin becomes oedematous and harsh. They may be isolated, but in 5% cases associated with Sturge–Weber syndrome. Ipsilateral angiomas of the meninges and brain can cause epileptic fits, hemoparesis, etc. Think of association with glaucoma in 30% ipsilateral to facial angioma. especially if upper eyelid involved.
26. **E** – Plexiform neurofibromas – association with NF-1.
27. **D** – Strawberry naevus tend to resolve with age, with 75% resolved by the age of four. Presentation 6–12 months. Remember deep lesions can present with proptosis. Rhabdomyosarcoma must be excluded (only with biopsy)!

Haemangioma of the eyelid: presents at adulthood spontaneously. Increases in size rapidly. Red-blood-filled cysts. Can be found in other parts of the body. A **pyogenic granuloma** can look similar but not blood filled and may have papillomatous appearance.

Theme: Lid abnormalities

28. **D** – Blepharophimosis syndrome: ptosis moderate to severe (symmetrical or slightly asymmetrical), telecanthus, epicanthus inversus, hypertelorism, lower lid ectropion, nasal bridge hypoplasia. Autosomal dominant inheritance.
29. **C**
30. **E**

Chapter 10: Neuro-ophthalmology Answers

Theme: Pupils I – mydriasis

1. **C**
2. **B**
3. **A** – Surgical trauma from multiple procedures.

Theme: Pupils II – miosis

4. **E**
5. **C**
6. **F**

Theme: Multiple cranial nerve palsies

7. **C**
8. **A** – Vestibular schwannomas are characteristic of neurofibromatosis 2.
9. **A**

Theme: Headache

10. **B** – Giant cell arteritis with an arteritic anterior ischaemic optic neuropathy.
11. **E**
12. **A**

Theme: Optic disc pallor

13. **D** – Disorder of maternal mitochondrial DNA.
14. **F** – Double ring sign = optic nerve hypoplasia, disc is surrounded by scleral ring and a ring of hyperpigmentation.
15. **A**

Theme: Phakomatoses

16. **B**
17. **E**
18. **D**

Theme: Facial nerve disorders

19. **E**
20. **A**
21. **C** – An abnormal synkinetic reflex causing orofacial dyskinesia.

Chapter 11: General Medicine Answers

Theme: Medical emergencies I

1. **F**
2. **C**
3. **D** – Anaphylaxis to intravenous fluorescein.

Theme: Treating medical emergencies

4. **D**
5. **B**
6. **F**

Theme: Brainstem syndromes that involve cranial nerves

7. **E**
8. **D**
9. **C**

Theme: Movement disorders

10. **E**
11. **D**
12. **B**

Theme: Spinal cord disorders

13. **E**
14. **F**
15. **C**

Theme: Peripheral sensory neuropathy

16. **B**
17. **F**
18. **D**